PRAISE FOR HIGH PERFORMANCE HEALTH

"If you are ready to seize the day and raise your health to the best level possible, this is your book. It's a blueprint for not just the body, but for the mind and spirit as well."

Larry Dossey, MD
Author, *The Extraordinary Healing Power of Ordinary Things*

"James Rippe is wise, loving, and reliable. *High Performance Health* is one of those truly rare books that is both eminently practical and deeply inspiring. If you want to live to your optimum health potential, you would have a hard time finding a better guide."

John Robbins
Author, *Healthy At 100* and *Diet For A New America*

"This book is a gem that challenges and inspires you to live your best life and health now. Written with deep insights and warmth, Dr. Rippe takes you on the journey to high performance health by providing the essential tools and steps. He inspires, motivates and empowers. And you really feel like, '*I can do this!*'"

Hans Diehl, DrHSc, MPH, FACN
Lifestyle Medicine Institute
Best-selling Author and Founder of CHIP

"With *High Performance Health*, Dr. James Rippe has achieved a remarkable feat: He has created a soaring inspirational platform for delivering his highly practical and important health and fitness advice. Readers will delight in his literary virtuosity as he trips nimbly through the insights into well-being of Thoreau, Aristotle, T.S. Eliot, *Star Wars'* Obi Wan Kenobi, and legendary NFL quarterback Joe Montana – not to mention scientists reporting in such revered publications as the *Journal of the American Medical Association*. This is a must read for those who need a rousing boost as they launch their own personal health and fitness program."

William Proctor
Co-Author, *Start Strong, Finish Strong* with
Dr. Kenneth H. Cooper and Dr. Tyler C. Cooper

"Not unlike the world of sports, competing at the top levels of global business requires extraordinary energy and endurance. Jim Rippe, for me and many other executives, has gone beyond monitoring my health to showing me how to get more living out of life and enjoy the ride even more."

Rick Goings
Chairman & CEO
Tupperware Brands Corporation

"The idea that we are what we think is becoming more accepted. It is time that we realize that we should raise our expectations in all areas of life in order to achieve a high performance level. This book allows us to understand the steps necessary to accomplish this fact. It is my belief that if every American would read this and apply it, not only would we be able to overcome such conditions as depression, anxiety, fear, but we would cease the constant need for supplementing what is not within our control. This book allows a person to take control of their life in a balanced, healthy, spiritual manner."

Dr. Gary Null
Author, *Power Aging* and *Get Healthy Now*

"Dr. James Rippe always raises the bar of performance inviting millions to follow his happy, often gleeful rush into living and working up near the peak. He created unique walking fitness charts, the first systematic data that changed walking from good intentions and a clumsy form of semi-running into a disciplined door to fitness. We all owe him a great deal. He is indeed the Father of the American Walking Movement. You'll have a delightful time reading this book."

T. George Harris
Editor, Media Technology
University of California, San Diego

"In the more than ten years that I have known Dr. Rippe, he has exemplified the lifestyle that he describes in *High Performance Health*. A busy father, physician, and husband, Jim is an effective and inspirational role model for the mantra, 'Always strive to be the best you can be.' By embracing the 10 step program, each of us has the opportunity to improve our lives—physically, mentally, and spiritually."

Karen Miller-Kovach
Chief Scientific Officer
Weight Watchers International, Inc.

"High Performance Health is a wonderful book written by a pioneering cardiologist describing a journey to help us take back our health. Following the clear, succinct steps presented by Dr. Rippe will enable readers to lead richer and fuller lives and to achieve their optimal health. Highly recommended!"

John P. Foreyt, Ph.D.
Behavioral Medicine Research Center
Baylor College of Medicine
Houston, TX

"If you have the inspiration, desire and intention to change your life and reclaim your health then this book can coach and guide you through the changes required to accomplish your goals. It is an excellent resource for creating change in your mind, body and spirit."

Bernie Siegel, MD
Author, *Love, Medicine & Miracles* and *Love, Magic & Mud Pies*

"If you are looking for focus, inspiration, and direction in achieving stellar health, Dr. Rippe's *High Performance Health* is a must-read. Dr. Rippe is the quintessential doctor and healer who has helped thousands of top executives and athletes transform their health. Now, you can, too!"

Ann Louise Gittleman, Ph.D.
New York Times best-selling author, *The Fat Flush Plan*

"Jim Rippe has written a terrific, inspiring primer on how we can consciously remake our health. But *High Performance Health* is more than a medical self-help book, it's a how-to manual on living a high-performance life."

Jeff Levin, Ph.D., M.P.H.
Author of *God, Faith, and Health*

"We can transform our lives and take charge of our destinies through our lifestyle choices. *High Performance Health* gives you the tools you need to harness the power of prevention. No one has done more than Dr. James Rippe to help others overcome barriers and achieve optimal health."

JoAnn E. Manson, MD, Dr PH
Chief of Preventive Medicine, Brigham and Women's Hospital
Professor of Medicine, Harvard Medical School

HIGH PERFORMANCE
HEALTH

HIGH PERFORMANCE
HEALTH

10 REAL-LIFE SOLUTIONS
TO REDEFINE YOUR HEALTH
AND REVOLUTIONIZE YOUR LIFE

JAMES M. RIPPE, MD

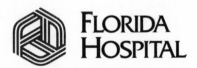

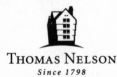

THOMAS NELSON
Since 1798

NASHVILLE   DALLAS   MEXICO CITY   RIO DE JANEIRO   BEIJING

Published in Nashville, TN, by Thomas Nelson. Thomas Nelson is a trademark of Thomas Nelson, Inc.

Published in association with the literary agency of Alive Communications, Inc., 7680 Goddard St., Suite 200, Colorado Springs, CO 80920.

Thomas Nelson, Inc. titles may be purchased in bulk for educational, business, fund-raising, or sales promotional use. For information, please e-mail SpecialMarkets@ThomasNelson.com.

Scripture quotations are taken from the New King James Version®. Copyright © 1982 by Thomas Nelson, Inc. Used by permission. All rights reserved.

AUTHOR'S NOTE: This book contains numerous case histories and patient stories. In order to preserve the privacy of the people involved, I have disguised their appearances, names, and personal stories so that they are not identifiable. Case histories may also include composite characters.

PUBLISHER'S NOTE: This book is not intended to replace a one-on-one relationship with a qualified health-care professional but is intended as a sharing of knowledge and information from the research and experience of the author. You are advised and encouraged to consult with your health-care professional in all matters relating to your health and the health of your family. The publisher and author disclaim any liability arising directly or indirectly from the use of this book.

General Editor, Florida Hospital: Todd Chobotar
Florida Hospital Review Board: Brian Paradis, Monica Reed, MD, Dick Tibbits, DMin
Photography: Spencer Freeman
Cover Design: Studio Gearbox – Chris Gilbert
Interior Design: Casey Hooper

Library of Congress Cataloging-in-Publication Data
Rippe, James M.
  High performance health : the 10-step mind, body & spirit program to revolutionize your life / James M. Rippe.
    p. cm.
  Includes bibliographical references and index.
  ISBN 978-0-8499-0182-9 (hardcover) 1. Physical fitness. 2. Exercise. 3. Health. 4. Mind and body. I. Title.

RA781.R5755 2007
613.7--dc22

                                                                        2006101159

Printed in the United States of America
07 08 09 10 11 QW 9 8 7 6 5 4 3 2 1

TO STEPHANIE, HART, JAELIN, DEVON, AND JAMIE

my reasons for living

And all shall be well and
All manner of things shall be well
When the tongues of flame are in-folded
Into the crowned knot of fire
And the fire and the rose are one.

—T. S. ELIOT
"Little Gidding"
The Four Quartets

CONTENTS

AUTHOR'S NOTE

Special thanks are due to Mary Abbott Waite. This is the sixth book-writing project on which Mary Abbott and I have collaborated. Mary Abbott is every writer's dream collaborator. She knows my voice, shares my values, has read the same books, and is committed to the same life journey that I am on. She took a very long, heartfelt, but sometimes rambling manuscript, polished the good points, discarded the bad, and shaped it into the final book that you see in front of you.

Mary Abbott has the rare gift of being able to disappear within an author's voice yet bring striking clarity and wisdom of her own without seeming to intrude. Without her absolute commitment to this journey, as well as her friendship, intelligence, and editorial skills, *High Performance Health* could never have happened.

ACKNOWLEDGMENTS

Clinical research, patient care, and book writing are all team sports. Or as the Beatles famously said, "I get by with a little help from my friends."

Over the years many incredible friends and colleagues in each of these areas have helped, supported, and taught me. To all those individuals too numerous to acknowledge by name, I am deeply grateful.

The clinical research I frequently refer to throughout this book has been conducted at Rippe Lifestyle Institute and Rippe Lifestyle Institute at Florida Hospital Celebration Health under the able direction of my great friend Ted Angelopoulos, PhD, MPH. Ted is the director of research at Rippe Lifestyle Institute and Rippe Health Assessment as well as professor of exercise science at the University of Central Florida, where he also serves at the research director for the Center for Lifestyle Medicine. Ted has inexhaustible energy and tremendous scientific skills. His friendship has been enormously important to me for many years.

Our associate director of research, Linda Zukley, MS, BS, RN, CCRN, is the only person I have ever met who can match the energy and enthusiasm of Dr. Angelopoulos. She not only has great clinical skills but is also a fantastic manager, with a deep dedication to all aspects of our clinical research at Rippe Lifestyle Institute. Ted and Linda are ably supported by a team of exercise physiologists, nutritionists, and other support staff, who do such a wonderful job carrying out the daily research that I often refer to in this book.

Amy Stachnik has done an outstanding job as director of client services for RHA and now plays a senior marketing role at the Florida Hospital Institute for Lifestyle Medicine. Page Heyward does a magnificent job of business development for the Florida Hospital Institute for Lifestyle Medicine.

My clinical facility, Rippe Health Assessment at Florida Hospital Celebration Health, and I are also blessed with a wonderful team of clinicians who deliver the high standard of clinical care and patient caring that are the hallmarks of the Rippe Health Assessment experience. The clinical team is led by Drs. Sherry Brooks and Sheri Novendstern, whose clinical skills and interpersonal skills inspire me every day. The daily clinical operations at Rippe Health Assessment are led by our clinic director, Herminio Alamo, MHA, RN, who leads the team of nurses, exercise physiologists, nutritionists, and support personnel that deliver a wonderful and caring clinical and personal experience to every patient every day at our clinic.

I am blessed to have Florida Hospital as my partner in both my clinic and now in a major clinical and research endeavor called the Florida Hospital Institute for Lifestyle Medicine (FHILM). Florida Hospital is the largest admitting hospital in America and is ably run by a team of senior executives who care passionately about, and deliver, the Florida Hospital mission to provide the "healing ministry of Christ." My friend and colleague, Brian Paradis, chief operating officer of Florida Hospital, has been a particularly important friend and mentor. Brian has supported my diverse efforts and helped me understand both spiritual and administrative aspects of health care. He also serves as chairman of the Florida Hospital Institute for Lifestyle Medicine. Lars Houmann, chief executive officer of Florida Hospital, has been a long-term supporter of our efforts at Rippe Health Assessment and the FHILM. Don Jernigan, the CEO of Adventist Health System, has been a staunch supporter in lifestyle medicine and executive health for many years. Dr. Des Cummings has inspired me with his creative ideas and served as a spiritual mentor for me. David Banks and Dr. Monica Reed have also guided me and supported our efforts at Florida Hospital.

Friends, professional colleagues, and mentors have also guided and helped me at various stages of my life and professional development. Dr. Joseph Alpert was an early and important mentor to me at Harvard Medical School and played a critical role in guiding me into a career in cardiology and research. Dr. Ira Ockene taught me how to do cardiac catheterization and served as a clinical mentor in all aspects of cardiology. Dr. Richard Irwin, who coedits a major intensive care medicine textbook with me (*Irwin and Rippe's Intensive Care Medicine*), has been a great friend, mentor, and role model.

Thanks to Todd Chobotar, director of publishing and creative productions at Florida Hospital, and Lee Hough, my literary agent on this project, who were early believers in the concept of this book. Acquisitions editor Debbie Wickwire has been a passionate and effective advocate, not only for the book but for the concept of high performance health from its earliest conception. Other executives at Thomas Nelson, including David Moberg and Jeff Loper, have also embraced and supported the concept of high performance health and this book project.

I am grateful for the numerous organizations and individuals who have sponsored key pieces of research that are discussed in the course of this book. Much of the research related to weight management would not have been possible without the support of the executive team at Weight Watchers, including its chairman, Ray Debbane; its CEO, Linda Heutt; the vice president of program development and chief scientific officer, Karen Miller Kovach, MS, RD; and board member Jonas Fajgenbaum. Issues related to technology and "early health" have been supported and clarified by my friend Joe Hogan, CEO of GE Healthcare. Other research colleagues include Nancy Green, PhD, RD;

Al Bolles, PhD; Lisa Carlson, MS, RD; Barbara Ivens, MS, RD; Mark Andon, PhD; and many others.

I have been fortunate to lead an academic effort at the University of Central Florida to establish the Center for Lifestyle Medicine at UCF. This would not have been possible without the strong support of the president of UCF, Dr. John Hitt, who is both a great friend and an advocate of the principles of lifestyle medicine and high performance health. Dick Nunis, the retired chairman of Walt Disney Attractions, Inc., chairman of the Board of Trustees at UCF, and godfather to my youngest child, has provided me with sage advice and support for many years.

I also want to acknowledge and thank my friend Joe Montana, who has been my partner in a major hypertension education campaign for five years and who wrote the foreword for this book. Joe is a true American hero who, in many ways, epitomizes both the personal and professional attributes of high performance health that I describe in this book.

The great physician Sir William Osler once said that to study medicine without books is the equivalent of going to sea without maps, but to study medicine without patients is to never go to sea at all. I am deeply grateful to the thousands of patients and research subjects who have come through our clinical research organization, Rippe Lifestyle Institute, and our clinic, Rippe Health Assessment, over the past two decades. They have taught me, inspired me, and touched my life in ways too numerous to count. I have used their stories liberally throughout this book but have changed their names and, in some instances, condensed experiences to illustrate important points and protect anonymity.

No project of this size and scope would be conceivable without my superb editorial director, Elizabeth Grady, who has directed all editorial activities for my organization for more than twenty years. Her fantastic organizational skills, enormous energy and commitment, and care for me and all of my diverse projects remain a great source of happiness and pride to me.

My executive assistant, Carol Moreau, flawlessly manages a complicated and busy career spanning many different aspects, including consulting, research, public speaking, and coordination of complex travel schedules. Carol unfailingly delivers the high level of performance and caring that epitomizes high performance health. Becky Cotton Hess, my executive assistant and coordinator for the Florida Hospital Institute for Lifestyle Medicine, and Debbie Rhodes, executive assistant at the University of Central Florida and coordinator of the Center for Lifestyle Medicine at UCF, support my efforts within those two organizations with great skill and caring.

My family has been a great source of comfort and support to me. My parents, Dr. Dayle Rippe and Elizabeth Rippe, now deceased, pushed me, loved me, and contributed to my growth as both a person and a parent in ways that I am only beginning to understand. My brothers, Dr. Richard Rippe and Dr. William Rippe, and their wives, Sandy and Marcia, and their children give me unfailing love and the support of a great family.

Finally, my dear wife, Stephanie Hart Rippe, has been my soul mate, inspiration, and constant source of love and support in all aspects of my life. I have sometimes thought that if I am the fire, then she is the rose. She inspires me with her beauty and commitment, not only to me but to our four fantastic daughters, Hart, Jaelin, Devon, and Jamie, who have brought more joy and meaning into my life than I ever thought possible. These five women, who together comprise the "Rippe women," endow my life with meaning and give me the strength and courage to continue on the path of high performance health that I have tried to outline in this book.

—JMR
Boston, Massachusetts

FOREWORD

Everyone wants to perform at his or her best. That was certainly my goal in 1979 when I was drafted as a quarterback by the San Francisco 49ers of the NFL. I thought I was pretty well prepared for what was ahead of me. I was coming from a great university, Notre Dame, with a great football program. We had won the National Championship in 1977. I had honed skills that I had been working on since my dad had first introduced me to the fundamentals. I trained hard. I was in great shape. How much more could I learn? Then I met my 49er teammates and Coach Bill Walsh.

At the NFL level, every athlete on my team and on opposing teams had talent and skill. Everyone had drive and determination. Everybody trained as hard as everybody else. As a result, every athlete was always looking for an edge, something that would push them to the next level. I was looking for that performance edge too. I found that the guys who consistently achieved peak performance were those who took the best care of themselves. That proved true for me. Taking care of my body and health, I think, gave me an edge for my whole career. When I really watched what I ate and drank and when I exerted the discipline to follow even stricter exercise guidelines than those used in training, I never felt better, and I was able to perform at my best even through long Super Bowl seasons. That lesson has carried over into the rest of my life and beyond my playing career.

Just as important, Bill Walsh, my coach and mentor, really taught me how to prepare with perfection in mind. He wanted us to complete 100 percent of our passes every day, from Monday's practice through Sunday's game. He really *worked* on that by paying attention to the little details of what was necessary. I don't know how many pro quarterbacks get taught the fundamentals of their position. But that's what we worked on. Bill Walsh knew that perfecting fundamentals such as my footwork, my body position, proper reads, and throwing the ball to the right person would help our team be successful. It didn't matter to him if it was a five-yard pass or a ninety-five-yard pass. A completion was a completion. He taught me that when things are going well, it's because you are executing the fundamentals, and when things are going badly, the only way to turn them around is to go back to the fundamentals. He felt that if you prepare with perfection in mind, then you will play with perfection in mind. That mind-set—and relentlessly practicing the fundamentals—took our 49ers team to four Super Bowl Championships.

What was true for performing at a high level as a professional athlete has carried over into my life as a businessman and in my family life. Performing at your best in any area of life requires taking care of yourself and making the most of your health. Performing at your best means mastering the fundamentals and putting them into play.

Helping you do that in your life is the goal of my friend Dr. James Rippe in *High Performance Health*. Jim's passionate about that. I've often heard him say, "Most people view good health as passive freedom from disease. They may smoke, be overweight, get little exercise, and have many major health risk factors, but as long as they can say, 'I'm not sick,' they rate their health as good or excellent. But your health can be so much more than that. Achieving your optimal health can be a springboard to high performance. It can be a springboard to achieving a richer, more meaningful life." In *High Performance Health*, Jim shows you how to take control of your health and turn it into a tool for achieving high performance. What you are holding in your hand is both a game plan and a playbook.

Jim and I first met about four years ago when we teamed up to lead a national public education campaign about high blood pressure. More than 65 million Americans have high blood pressure. Many don't know it. Although I stayed in condition after I retired from football, when I was forty six, I discovered that I had high blood pressure during a regular annual physical. My physician sent me right to a cardiologist. Together we worked in partnership to help me control my high blood pressure and lower my risk of heart disease, which runs in my family. For me, taking control has required making some simple changes in my diet and exercise habits and finding the right medication. Taking control has had the added benefit of helping me regain that performance edge for working and living. So I know what Jim Rippe is talking about when he urges you to take back responsibility for your health. He and I share the conviction that this is one of the most important things you can do for yourself and your family. We've shared this message all over the country over the last four years as our campaign has taken us to more than 50 cities, about 150 satellite interviews, and countless personal appearances, seminars, and media interviews.

Another part of the message is that if you are going to take control of your health and make it a tool for living more fully, then you will need a support team. Nobody achieves high performance all by themselves. Without the supportive partnerships and teams I enjoyed from my earliest days, for example, I could never have played football at the level I did. Early on, my father taught me the fundamentals of sports, and both of my parents gave me the example of discipline. In high school, college, and certainly the NFL, I had coaches who worked with me on skills and execution, and teammates who had the same competitive drive to excellence that I did. With the 49ers and Chiefs, I was successful because I had a bunch of great guys around me who had the same motives and goals, worked hard, and—so crucial—really enjoyed our time together. My greatest partnership is with my wife, Jennifer, who has been from day one my best friend. Playing highly competitive pro football is all-consuming. You are away from home a lot; you have to deal with injuries and huge pressures. When things were tough for me then, when things are tough now, Jennifer is always there. She continues to set the example for me in our most challenging and important job—raising our family of four children. In this book, Jim Rippe shows you how to build the personal partnerships and support team that can help you achieve your goals for health and high performance.

In this foreword, it's been a pleasure to share with you from my experience a few thoughts about what's required to perform at your best, whatever the task or goal. Three keys for me are

- taking care of yourself in order to maximize your health,
- taking personal responsibility for your health and performance, and
- building supportive partnerships and enjoying them.

As I said earlier, Dr. James Rippe's *High Performance Health* provides you both a game plan and a playbook for achieving your best health and your best performance. As a cardiologist and research scientist, Jim Rippe has worked with elite performers and ordinary people from all walks of life to help them achieve better health and fuller lives. As a human being, husband, and father of four, he has put the principles of high performance health to work in his own life. I know, because we've often shared "war stories." In *High Performance Health*, he shares what you need to know—the science, the techniques, the insights and wisdom, and many inspiring individual stories. You'll even find a few stories about one Joe Montana. So I challenge you to open the book and take the first steps to achieving your own goals for high performance health.

—Joe Montana
San Francisco, California

PART 1 | DIAGNOSIS AND UNDERSTANDING

1 | YOU WILL PROTECT WHAT YOU LOVE

What thou lovest well remains,
the rest is dross.
  —EZRA POUND, *THE CANTOS*

There is a land of the living and a land of the dead
and the bridge is love, the only survival, the only meaning.
  —THORNTON WILDER, *THE BRIDGE OF SAN LUIS REY*

Who do you love? Your family? Your friends and neighbors? Yourself?

The willingness to protect what we love is so fundamental that it seems to be wired into our DNA. Consider this: What parent wouldn't lay down his or her own life to save a child? I know this to be true from personal experience. My wife and I have been blessed with four daughters, and if any of them were in danger, I would willingly give my life to ensure safety. It's a simple fact: what you love, you will protect.

Do you love yourself and your family enough to protect your health? If you are like most people, your answer is a resounding "Yes!" This is a book about how to achieve the best life possible by protecting and renewing a precious asset many of us have taken for granted or simply misunderstood: good health.

In the chapters that follow, you will learn how to view your health in a whole new way—as the springboard to a joyful, dynamic, and meaningful life.

HOW DO YOU VIEW YOUR HEALTH?

Every two years, the U.S. Department of Health and Human Services asks American adults to rate their health on a scale from poor to excellent. Do you think most of us regard ourselves as in poor health or in good health? The answer may surprise you. Consistently, more than 90 percent of respondents rate their health as either "good" or "excellent."

It's a simple fact: what you love, you will protect.

Let's consider this perception. More than 90 percent of us report our health is good. But the number of Americans who have risk factors for chronic diseases or who engage in risky behaviors tells a very different story:

- In the U.S., more than 66 percent of adults are overweight or obese.[1]
- Despite decades of warnings about cigarette smoking, about one out of every four men and one out of every five women in the United States still smoke cigarettes.[2]
- More than 70 percent of adults do not exercise enough to achieve health benefits, and 40 percent of adults are truly sedentary.[3]
- Fewer than 25 percent of adults consume the recommended number of servings of fruits and vegetables on a regular basis.[4]
- When it comes to the key behaviors that could eliminate 80 percent of heart disease, the number one killer of both men and women in the United States, as few as a dismal

3 percent of adults may follow all of these simple daily health practices.[5]

How can we square these grim statistics with the fact that more than 90 percent of adults view their health as good or excellent? The most convincing explanation I can come up with is that most people view their health as simply the *passive freedom from disease*. In other words, if you feel okay today, that's good enough; don't worry about the future.

Of course, being free from disease is an important place to start, but health can be much more than that. Health can be a springboard for achieving a joyous, dynamic, and meaningful life. This is what I mean by "high performance health"—using your health as a tool that enables you to accomplish things you've only dreamed about.

You may think high performance health is only for high-level executives or professional athletes. Not so! Let me say clearly that high performance health is within your grasp. *High performance health* means achieving your best health now. Achieving your best health includes defining your values, setting goals based on those values, and using them to live to your highest potential physically, mentally, and spiritu-

> High performance health means achieving your best health now.

ally. As a result, your best health in turn becomes the springboard to many other benefits. In this book, I will share how you can achieve these benefits in your own life through simple daily practices.

KNOWLEDGE IS NOT ENOUGH

When it comes to achieving high performance health as an active springboard to a fulfilling life, many of us struggle to connect what we know about how to maximize our health with what we actually do daily. Let me give you a telling example.

In 2000, Meir Stampfer and colleagues published a major study on heart disease and women in the prestigious *New England Journal of Medicine*. (Note: Heart disease is the leading cause of death for women and kills more women than men annually.) This study was based on the landmark Nurses' Health Study, which followed more than eighty-four thousand female nurses for fourteen years. After examining all the data from this study, the authors concluded that 80 percent of all heart attacks and/or heart disease deaths in women could be attributed to failure to follow a low-risk pattern of lifestyle practices, such as not smoking, maintaining a healthy body weight, following a few simple nutritional practices, and obtaining thirty minutes of physical activity on most days. Imagine the power of these simple practices to eliminate many cases of the leading cause of death in women! Yet only 3 percent of the nurses in this study followed all five of these practices, and only 7 percent followed four practices.[6] And remember, these are health-care workers who should know better.

Clearly, knowledge alone is not enough to change the way we think about our health. As one of my physician colleagues observed, "Everyone who smokes knows they shouldn't, and everyone who doesn't exercise knows they should!" For this reason, I am not going to spend much time telling you to eat better, lose weight, or exercise. Of course, all these things are beneficial, and in Chapter 3 I will give you some practical tips and techniques you may find helpful. But you already know what you ought to do. If achieving positive change were as simple as being aware that you should exercise more and eat better, you would have done that a long time ago.

Instead, I am going to ask you to join me in a simpler and more important journey to view your health in a fundamentally different way—as an essential value for high performance living. Then you can use that understanding as a springboard to change.

A PERSONAL JOURNEY

Before you begin your journey toward high performance health, I'd like to share something of my own journey with you. The concept of high performance health has grown into an effective and practical strategy over many years as I worked as a physician and medical researcher. My views of medicine, health, and healing evolved as I discovered more about the science of lifestyle medicine and its grounding in strong mind-body-spirit connections and values.

When I started my medical training at Harvard Medical School in 1975, I believed in fitness. I was an avid runner/jogger and ran forty-five miles a week. I had played both high-school and college sports. After college, I earned my black belt in karate by working out at least an hour a day for three years. With my interests in fitness and athletic conditioning, cardiology was a natural fit for me. By the time I was a second-year medical student, I was totally enamored of the heart and everything that had to do with it. After four years at medical school and two years of internship and residency at Massachusetts General Hospital, one of the toughest residency programs in the United States, I finished my cardiology training with a three-year fellowship at the University of Massachusetts Medical School.

When I emerged from this intensive training, I felt confident in my ability to handle virtually any aspect of cardiovascular medicine. Somebody once said that if you are trained as a hammer, you see the world as a nail. Over nine years, I had been completely trained as a high-tech "hammer," and for a brief—and in retrospect, unfortunate—time in my life, I viewed my patients as "nails." I was determined to apply all of my hard-won knowledge and technical skills in the treatment of cardiovascular disease. I even specialized in the most high-tech aspect of cardiology and spent the first ten years of my professional life as an academic cardiologist performing thousands of heart catheterizations and training cardiology fellows to do this complicated procedure.

Slowly, however, it began to dawn on me that something was wrong with this approach. Certainly we were saving lives, but I was beginning to feel very much like the man in the old story who lived by the river and spent all day pulling drowning people out of the water. After rescuing multitudes, the man finally decided to walk up the river and find out who was pushing the victims in. I was also struck by how many of my patients came back to me again and again either unwilling or unable to change the habits that got them into trouble in the first place. I decided that there had to be a better way to prevent and treat heart disease that would help more patients avoid the cath lab, angioplasties, and heart surgeries.

> If I was going to make a difference, I had to help my patients take better care of themselves.

So I founded an exercise physiology laboratory at the University of Massachusetts Medical School, and we started doing research. Ultimately we explored fitness walking as an activity to help people gain control of their lives and lower their risk of cardiovascular disease. This research led to a series of publications and books, as well as the first walking test for people to estimate their cardiovascular fitness. As a result of this work, I received the designation "father of the American walking movement," a designation I am extremely proud of.

While I was passionately involved in helping my patients and pursuing research, however, subtle changes—not for the better—were slipping up on me personally. During my internship and residency, for instance, I gained weight for the first time in my life. I was a prisoner to the long hours, stress, and fatigue of being a house officer (resident). I found it impossible to maintain a regular exercise program. I snagged meals when and as I could, often from the vending machine. I gained fifteen or twenty pounds. The natural energy I'd always enjoyed seemed submerged in a rolling fog of fatigue. Something had to change for me, as well as for my patients, if I was going to realize my calling as a physician to enable health and healing.

These and many other factors convinced me that if I was going to make a difference, I had to help my patients take better care of themselves. And I had to do the same for myself. To do that, I realized that I had to stop being a high-tech "hammer" and become a different kind of partner with my patients. Please don't get me wrong; I still have enormous admiration for the technical aspects of medicine and cardiology. These advanced tools have an important role to play in total health, but they need to be used in the context of supporting health as a dynamic springboard to wholeness, not simply as treatment to produce the passive absence of disease.

My passion for health continues to grow as I work with hundreds of people like you. And so does my personal perspective. Becoming a husband and father, for example, has deepened my passion for health as a life-giving value. In the early 1990s, I married the woman of my dreams, and as I mentioned earlier, we have been blessed with four beautiful daughters. I want to be at my best for each of these wonderful "Rippe women" today and tomorrow and for thousands of tomorrows thereafter. As you would expect, this personal experience and commitment has helped my view of high performance health to change, evolve, and deepen.

> I promise you will find the high performance approach to health fresh and empowering.

I tell you these things because I want you to know that as we work together through this book, I'm sharing from deep personal conviction as well as medical expertise. Based on my personal experience and that of the many patients I've worked with, I promise you will find the high performance approach to health fresh and empowering.

LIFESTYLE MEDICINE: THE POWER OF DAILY HABITS

Hundreds, if not thousands, of scientific studies support the concept that our daily habits have a profound impact on our health and quality of life. This link between daily actions and health is called *lifestyle medicine.*

I became interested in this area for two reasons. First, an extensive body of medical literature reported overwhelming evidence that such habits and actions as physical activity, nutritional choices, weight management, and smoking have a significant impact on health. But the medical community in general was not doing much to explore how they might be used to promote health and prevent chronic diseases. Second, the burgeoning popularity of numerous "alternative" nutrition, fitness, and health practices indicated that Americans are eager for advice or regimens to enhance health and wellness, but too often they turn to scientifically unproven and even highly dubious practices and products whose promoters typically promise "miraculous," "overnight" changes and benefits, often with "no work on your part."

As a result of my concern, I established one of the first research laboratories and clinics in lifestyle medicine. In the last twenty years, the research organization and clinic have become the world leaders in the area of lifestyle medicine.

> One of the essentials of high performance health is that it is based on valuing good health as a precious trust that yields enormous rewards when protected and enhanced.

At the Rippe Lifestyle Institute in Massachusetts and Florida, we have presented and published more than three hundred academic papers on topics ranging from stress reduction to nutrition, weight management, and fitness and their impact on disease prevention and management. Thousands of research volunteers from all walks of life have come through our laboratory to benefit from these research studies and to change their lives for the better.

The Rippe Health Assessment clinic at the Florida Hospital Institute of Lifestyle Medicine Celebration Health has used the principles of lifestyle medicine to help thousands of patients achieve high performance health. Our approach is very simple: we combine the best of modern medical and surgical techniques with a firm emphasis on lifestyle practices and the need for physicians and patients to form partnerships to achieve the best outcomes. Every patient leaves our clinic with a detailed plan for how he or she can change lifestyle practices to improve overall health.

I tell you all this to let you know that you are not alone. Over many years of work, we have had the opportunity to learn from thousands of patients and volunteers. I am grateful for their participation with us and proud to share with you their stories of how they have used the principles of lifestyle medicine to change their health for the better.

A VALUES-BASED APPROACH TO HEALTH

One of the essentials of high performance health is that it is based on valuing good health as a precious trust that yields enormous rewards when protected and enhanced. In this values-based approach, health is just one core value in a series of interrelated values that affect not only our physical health but also our quality of life and spiritual well-being. The figure below represents these *high performance health values.*

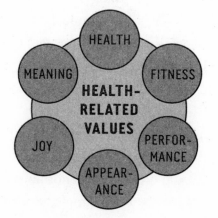

As you can see, this circle of values links the concepts of health, fitness, performance, appearance, joy, and meaning. Each value plays a vital role in achieving high performance health as a springboard to high performance living. Each helps us link health to our daily actions. Here's a brief overview.

Health. Health is at the top of the circle because it's our main focus of this book. Health in a larger sense means achieving your optimal physical, mental, and spiritual well-being.

Fitness. By fitness, I don't just mean physical fitness. I mean the capacity to meet or exceed the challenges you face in daily life, such as having the energy to take care of your children or grandchildren. Sound health strategies, such as regular medical care, physical activity, and even nutritional balance, fit into this concept as we fuel our bodies to perform at their best. Spiritual fitness and connectedness to others are also key components of this view of fitness.

Performance. Performance is the daily excellence you put into practice to achieve your goals as well as to meet the challenges life puts in front of you. Although performance has a distinct individual slant, it also has some universal qualities. My friend Joe Montana once told me that San Francisco 49ers coach Bill Walsh instructed his players never to walk on the football field without thinking of perfection, even if it was in practice, because ultimately performance rests on daily actions and habits. Or as Aristotle famously said, "We are what we repeatedly do. Excellence, then, is not an act, but a habit." In this book, I will give you a set of principles, practices, and habits that can turn your health into a powerful performance tool for living the way you desire.

Appearance. By appearance, I don't mean physical beauty. The excessive emphasis our culture places on physical beauty warps our understanding of true beauty and often causes enormous heartache as people pursue unrealistic body images. For example, in the privacy of my medical office, senior executives have asked me how they can get "six-pack abs." The answer is that they can't and probably shouldn't even if they could. The bodybuilders on the late-night infomercials for various abdominal machines often spend four to five hours a day exercising and have often stripped their body fat to unhealthy levels.

Rather, what I mean by appearance is the irresistible attractiveness we find in people who are engaging and full of life. All of us know individuals who may not possess physical beauty and yet are a joy to be with and demonstrate great energy, vitality, and presence. If you put into place the principles I describe in this book, your friends will ask you, "What are you doing? You look great!" Your good health, better health than you have ever felt before, will radiate vitality.

Joy. Good health can be a source of joy in your life, and joy and happiness in turn can contribute to good health. There is a powerful relationship between your mind and emotions and your body. Numerous studies have shown the important role of emotions in health and healing. In Chapter 5 we will look at the importance of creating a positive mental environment and of finding joy in order to achieve high performance health.

Meaning. When was the last time you thought about your health as a source of meaning? Yet living a life of meaning and purpose is not only a worthy goal to pursue but is vital to high performance health. Good health should be a source of meaning and purpose in all of our lives. Conversely, if we are able to find meaning in our lives, it will contribute in significant ways to our overall good health.

HOW TO USE THIS BOOK

As you begin your life-changing journey toward high performance health, let me say a few words about how to use this book. The book is divided into two parts. Part 1, "Diagnosis and Understanding," guides you through the fundamental principles we have developed that have helped thousands of people master the principles of high performance health. We will talk about how you can achieve your best health now by mastering the basics, building a high performance health team, transforming your life through high performance thinking, overcoming the barriers to high performance health, and using this concept as a springboard to high performance living. Because I want you to do a lot of thinking and planning as you read through these chapters, I have given you some basic assignments at the end of each chapter, called "Making It Personal."

Part 2, "Action Plan," is much shorter in length but just as important as Part 1. Over the years, I have learned the importance of giving people a simple yet specific plan for applying the principles of high performance health. Part 2 provides a step-by-step guide to putting into practice the principles of high performance health, as well as some encouragement drawn from my own journey of high performance health.

> **With this book, I invite you to take my hands, and together we will explore the exciting and powerful concept of high performance health.**

Throughout the book, I will share stories with you. Some of these are performance stories that draw on the lessons learned by individuals who changed their lives by mastering the principles of high performance health. Others are healing stories that touch on the lives, hopes, and aspirations of people who overcame health challenges by learning to work with, rather than against, their bodies' own healing power. I also share stories from my own personal experience.

The book also draws on the research and clinical practice we have accumulated during the last twenty years by treating thousands of patients and research subjects, in addition to wider medical literature. Where appropriate, I will help you separate the proven from the speculative or unproven. Throughout the process, I ask you to be my partner, since it is only through this type of partnership that we can achieve the best outcome.

TAKE MY HANDS—AND TAKE BACK YOUR HEALTH

As a physician, I have often thought that one of the failings of our medical system is that we often don't emphasize the importance of human touch by telling our patients, "Take my hands. Together we can do this." So with this book, I invite you to take my hands, and together we will explore the exciting and powerful concept of high performance health.

Each of us has enormous power to be the primary change-agent of our own health. Sure, there are wonderful things that modern medicine can do for you, but achieving high performance health depends first and foremost on your taking responsibility for yourself.

So join me in the quest to take back your health. I am not asking you to turn your life upside down, but I will be asking you to stop and take stock of what you are doing right now and what you can do to improve your health every day.

I'm reminded of the bridge that Thornton Wilder described in his famous novel, *The Bridge of San Luis Rey*, that divides "the land of the living and the land of the dead." That bridge is *love*. Love is the bridge to life. What you love, you will protect. Today, as you start this book, I ask you to hold my hand and walk across that bridge to the living land of high performance health. I'll be your guide to help you implement the ideas and techniques that work best for you. As you move from viewing good health as simply the absence of disease to understanding it as a fundamental gift from God, you will grow to see good health as a precious trust that yields enormous rewards when protected and enhanced. The difference those concepts can make in your life is nothing less than revolutionary.

2 | ACHIEVE YOUR BEST HEALTH NOW

We shall not cease from exploration
And the end of all our exploring
Will be to arrive where we started
And know the place for the first time.

  —T. S. ELIOT, "LITTLE GIDDING," *THE FOUR QUARTETS*

In the bulb there is a flower; in the seed, an apple tree;
in cocoons, a hidden promise: butterflies will soon be free!
In the cold and snow of winter there's a spring that waits to be,
unrevealed until its season, something God alone can see.

  —NATALIE SLEETH, "HYMN OF PROMISE"

What will it take to achieve your best health now? The journey to high performance health starts with assessing your story—what has gone on and is going on in your life. As you examine your story, what do you need to know to progress toward turning your health into a springboard for dynamic living?

My patient Frank had answered that fundamental question before he arrived for his first evaluation. At seventy-eight years old, Frank was a lean, intense man. Two devastating heart attacks had severely weakened his heart. Where each normal heartbeat pumps about 75 percent of the blood the heart holds, Frank's heart pumped only 15 to 20 percent. This condition leads to congestive heart failure. Because of the heart's weak output (the "failure"), blood tends to back up in the lungs (the "congestion"), causing shortness of breath and other difficulties. I told Frank his condition was extremely serious.

> The journey to high performance health starts with assessing your story

Undaunted, Frank was determined to get as much out of his remaining time as possible. That meant he was not giving up the twenty-acre peach orchard he had lovingly tended for more than fifty years. His wife, Myrtle, a sprightly woman in her seventies and a retired nurse, was determined to help in Frank's care so he could continue doing things he found enjoyable and meaningful.

I adjusted Frank's medicines to give his heart a boost and take some pressure off his lungs. But sadly, I knew that despite optimizing his medical regimen, and even if he weren't already seventy-eight, Frank at best had only about a 10 percent chance of surviving for five years because of the damage that had already occurred to his heart.

I continued to see Frank every three to six months and could always count on Frank and Myrtle bringing me a basket of peaches from their orchard in season. Frank continued to actively tend his beloved orchard for the next seven or eight years. He finally retired to a more supervisory role. He died peacefully, surrounded by his family, ten years after I met him. His funeral was attended by hundreds of friends who had gotten to know him over the years, either from buying his peaches or from participating with him in church or civic organizations.

Why did Frank beat the odds by living twice as long as the most optimistic prediction? Certainly the changes he made in the basics, such as nutrition, rest, and exercise, played a role. But they may not have been the most important factors. I believe Frank's survival hinged on several critical attributes of high performance health.

Frank was an optimist, the ultimate in high performance thinking. He looked forward with expectation, not fear or dread. Like farmers and gardeners, orchardists are by their very nature optimists. Each year they plant seeds or young plants and tend their growth. They learn to work with nature and not against it. They learn to plan for the unexpected (like the weather) and then to accept whatever happens. Each year they enjoy seeing the fruits of their labors. I think the exercise Frank derived from his work in the orchard may have contributed to his physical conditioning, but mostly he got the spiritual benefit of his optimism, his love of the land, and his forward-looking purpose.

Frank also had other pluses going for him, particularly the connection, love, and support of his wife and friends. Just as he tended his orchard, he also tended his marriage and his friendships. He was a man who gave and accepted love. Growing the best peaches for others was just one way he had of sharing love.

What does this have to do with achieving high performance health? After all, Frank had *severe* heart disease. Certainly, Frank faced many challenges. But while his heart was weakened, his spirit never flagged. I was impressed by his determination and optimism and his fervent belief that he could achieve his best health every day. There is no doubt in my mind that Frank doubled his survival because of these attributes. Freedom from disease was denied Frank, but he certainly used his best health now as a springboard for living.

WHAT WILL IT TAKE TO ACHIEVE YOUR BEST HEALTH NOW?

What can you do to achieve not just good health but your best health now? The good news is that you can achieve the health your body was designed for. In this chapter, we begin to discover your personal path to high performance health.

Many patients who come to our clinic ask how they can achieve their best health now. Some are simply seeking reassurance that they do not have a life-threatening disease. We do our best to provide that reassurance, but we also ask our patients to explore wider possibilities. We ask about their values and their goals. By the time patients leave our clinic, they are no longer simply seeking good health. They know their health can be the springboard to high performance living, and each person leaves with a plan geared to the realities of their life, their current health status, and their goals.

> The good news is that you can achieve the health your body was designed for.

In this chapter, we'll look at important concepts you need to achieve your best health now. More details will come in subsequent chapters, as we delve deeply into the techniques and understandings that my team and I have derived over many years of research and clinical practice.

IDENTIFYING THE KEYS TO ACHIEVING HIGH PERFORMANCE HEALTH

In *The Four Quartets*, the great twentieth-century poet T. S. Eliot, musing on the human spirit, wrote, "We shall not cease from exploration / And the end of all our exploring / Will be to arrive where we started / And know the place for the first time."[1] If we want our lives to have purpose and meaning, I think that "exploring" and continuing to seek and grow are essential. Most of us "started" with good health and energy. One of the goals of exploring the possibilities of high performance health is that you will arrive at a new understanding and knowledge of this great gift—and that you will be able to use this gift as the Creator intended.

Whether you enjoy basically good health or have health challenges as severe as Frank's, you can take steps right now to make your health better tomorrow than it is today. You can achieve high performance health. From Frank's experience we can identify several important keys to achieving high performance health. Just as they were within Frank's grasp, they are also within yours.

ASSESSING YOUR HISTORY—PHYSICAL, EMOTIONAL, AND SPIRITUAL. We have seen that the journey toward high performance health starts with a question: What is your story? We are all fascinated by stories and often learn from them. In medicine, we are particularly interested in a special version of your story that we call your "medical history." In fact, you're probably better acquainted than you would like with all those forms that you have to arrive half an hour early to fill out before a doctor's appointment.

Every health evaluation we perform at Rippe Health Assessment starts with assembling and assessing a patient's complete personal health profile (or "story"). In addition to asking about health conditions past and present, medications, family history, and any current concerns or complaints, we also ask each person to tell us about daily activities and habits that might promote health or put it at risk. These lifestyle attributes include such things as what and how they eat, how active they are, the quality of their sleep and rest, whether they smoke, their alcohol consumption patterns, and the like. But in many ways the most important part of getting to know the patient is asking him or her to share areas of satisfaction and dissatisfaction in personal life, work, and relationships; to evaluate the impact of stress in these same areas; and to describe other aspects of their environment and what makes them tick. And we never forget to ask, "What are your hopes, dreams, and aspirations?"

> You can take steps right now to make your health better tomorrow than it is today.

When Frank came to me for specialist evaluation and care, he had already learned as much as he could about his condition, and he had thought deeply about how he wanted to approach his future. With Myrtle's support, he was ready to dig more deeply into his options and possibilities and strategize to make the most of his physical strengths (and what I saw as his mental and spiritual strengths) so he could live as fully as he intended.

Later in the chapter, I will give you an assignment to help you begin to assess where you are and what you want to accomplish. But this is just the starting point for more important steps.

MASTERING THE BASICS. I promised not to nag you about the daily activities and practices that you know you ought to incorporate into your life in order to promote health and well-being. But everyone can use a review and useful new insights from the latest research studies.

Frank and Myrtle knew many of the basics of appropriate nutrition, physical activity, stress management, and the like, but they continued to learn, to adapt good strategies to Frank's needs, and to incorporate new ideas. In the next chapter, I will share how both high performance athletes and ordinary folks have tapped into the power of these dynamic tools and give you an overview of how to use them in your personal health journey.

IDENTIFYING AND STRENGTHENING SUPPORTIVE PARTNERSHIPS. High performance health is not achieved in a vacuum. Frank had a Rock-of-Gibraltar support in Myrtle, and I like to think I was a pretty steady influence in his life too. Beyond his wife and physician, Frank had important and deep connections with family and friends in the community, in his church, and in valued civic activities.

No matter where you live or how you currently assess your health, you can become the captain of your own high performance health team. Chapter 4 explores the important concepts and the many resources at your command.

TAPPING INTO HIGH PERFORMANCE THINKING AND MIND-BODY-SPIRIT CONNECTIONS. The most important qualities that Frank had going for him were his high performance thinking and his grounded spiritual strengths. In working with thousands of people who have been striving to build better health, I have observed that the major stumbling blocks to success are not anchored in challenges posed by nutritional changes or an exercise program or other aspects of their action plan. Instead, the major stumbling blocks are anchored in feelings and attitudes and in a personal sense of worthiness or unworthiness.

> High performance health is not achieved in a vacuum.

Frank did not have much to work with physically after the damage of two major heart attacks. But he had the most important qualities in huge measure. His strengths were rooted in his values, philosophical outlook, and faith. Here are just four of the strengths that empowered Frank:

- *He had let go of guilt.* When you have a major health challenge as Frank did, perhaps one that you know personal choices (such as smoking or being overweight) contributed to, it's easy to blame yourself and to feel guilty. But guilt is a quicksand trap—it will engulf you and destroy you. Using the best scientific understanding then available, Frank let me look carefully at what might be contributing to his heart condition and plan necessary changes; then he set his face forward. Part of letting go of guilt is forgiving yourself for what is and then going forward.

- *Frank accepted that he was worthy of the gift of life.* A man of faith, Frank believed deeply in God's reconciling love and grace, and he was assured that he was worthy of the Creator's love and acceptance. Living as fully and purposefully as possible is the best way of affirming and responding to God's love and acceptance.

- *Frank kept looking forward, planning, and exploring.* Frank didn't dwell in the past or on "what might have beens"; he planned for the future and kept exploring and living forward.

- *Frank lived one day at a time*. Although Frank and Myrtle had what we would call a "strategic plan" for extending Frank's future as far as possible, they lived one day at a time. Frank enjoyed each day's tasks, challenges, interactions with friends, gifts, laughs, and fulfillments. He didn't just stop to smell the peach blossoms; he lived at a pace that allowed him to receive and appreciate whatever each day had to offer, and when he needed to retreat to rest, he did.

Starting with Chapter 4 and continuing throughout the rest of the book, we explore many aspects of how achieving high performance health means drawing on all aspects of body, mind, and spirit.

PLANNING GOALS AND ADOPTING STRATEGIES TO ACCOMPLISH THEM. In my experience with thousands of patients, a major factor that separates the individuals who are able to move forward into high performance health and those who are not is the ability to plan. After all, if you don't know where you're starting and you don't have a plan for where you are going, it is unlikely that you'll end up at your goal.

My monitoring and adjusting Frank's medications was one way of supporting his plan for better health. Together we also looked at other steps he could take with diet and at how to judge his level of physical activity so he could determine when he was crossing the line from beneficial to overdoing. Frank's plans didn't turn his life upside down, and I'm not asking you to do that or to change everything at once. Rather, as

> A major factor that separates the individuals who are able to move forward into high performance health and those who are not is the ability to plan.

you work with me through this book, we'll look carefully at aspects of your health and help you plan the incremental steps that fit your life and help you move from your current health to your best health.

DISCOVERING YOUR PURPOSE SO THAT YOU CAN LIVE ON PURPOSE. When he entered my office the first time, Frank already knew that continuing to nurture his orchard was a cornerstone of meaning in his life. It's taken other people I've worked with a little longer.

Fran, a publishing executive, first came to our clinic when she was in her late thirties. She had started smoking in her early twenties, partly because cigarettes occupied her hands during long hours of evaluating manuscripts, and the nicotine buzz seemed to boost her alertness. As an editor of health books, she certainly knew that smoking elevated her risks for heart disease and cancer. She wanted badly to kick the habit. But smoking is highly addictive. For years, every time I saw Fran, we discussed various strategies for quitting—nicotine patches, support groups, psychotherapy, and many other options. But none she adopted worked long-term.

> The God-given purpose for good health is so that we can live at our best, realize our full potential, and truly enjoy our lives and the people we love and the purposes we were called to fulfill.

Then one year, she proudly announced herself as a "former" smoker. "What finally worked?" I asked. She smiled as she responded, "I focused my self-interest. My children were about to enter college, to start their adult lives, and I realized how much I wanted to be around to see their success and, most important, to see my grandchildren." Fran had discovered a purpose that was more compelling and motivating than future personal risk. She had also identified a strategy that would work for her. "I recognized that I needed to substitute one addiction for another. I started walking and within a few weeks was able to crumple up my last pack of cigarettes and throw them away for good. I am now walking four miles a day and have never felt better in my life." Ten years later, Fran is still off cigarettes and has two beautiful grandchildren she lavishes time on when she is not continuing her career at the highest levels of publishing.

I believe that the God-given purpose for good health is so that we can live at our best, realize our full potential, and truly enjoy our lives and the people we love and the purposes we were called to fulfill. Lasting change doesn't happen unless you can tap into your deeply held values—values that speak to your soul, telling you who you are, why you are here, and where you belong.

AFFIRMING THE MIRACLE OF LIFE. While we're thinking about health and living on purpose, I want us to pause and contemplate how miraculous our life and health really are—particularly our bodies, the structures that house life and health, mind and spirit.

Let me give you an example from my own field of cardiology. Consider the human heart and cardiovascular system. Every day, our hearts beat sixty to seventy times a minute, more than one hundred thousand times a day, more than three million times a year. This small, muscular organ, a little larger than the size of a clenched fist and weighing less than a pound, pumps five quarts of blood throughout our bodies every minute but is capable of increasing that output eight-fold during heavy exertion. All of this is designed to supply oxygen and nutrients to every organ, muscle, and other tissue in our bodies. Three little arteries, approximately the diameter of a pencil, supply our hearts with an uninterrupted flow of oxygen. The heart performs an elaborate dance with the entire cardiovascular system, which is capable of dilating and contracting to accept blood and squeeze it through the body. All of this takes place second by second, minute by minute, hour by hour in the unending miracle of life.

The same elegant complexity can be found in our nervous system, which controls virtually every action and thought that we have, in our lungs, our kidneys, our gastrointestinal tracts, and every organ system in our bodies. These are divine gifts that we have been given at birth, and it is our job to use them, protect them, and cherish them so that they can do the tasks they were designed to accomplish. The goal of high performance health is to give you the tools and motivation to guard these precious assets and to maximize their health and function.

YOU ARE WORTHY

If the actions and behaviors that support excellent health and the ability to live and perform at one's best are not in themselves complicated or difficult, why do so many of us have such a hard time starting a plan for change, much less carrying that plan through to long-term success?

The main barrier, in my experience, comes from within: deep down many of us don't think we are worthy of success or "worth taking the trouble for." This isn't just an issue of how we view our health, either. Such self-doubt or sense of unworthiness touches almost everyone's life, including my own. Growing up in a family that prized the highest achievement in academics and sports, I achieved—and too often I wondered if I was loved for myself or because of my achievements. Those doubts, buried inside, lingered into adulthood until the love of my wonderful wife and children convinced me that I truly was worthy and could be and was loved for myself and not for what I did.

In the face of self-doubt, we must open ourselves up to the miracle of God's gift of life and love. Just because you are a human being created by God, you are worthy not only of life but of the best life you can achieve. You are worthy and valuable for yourself alone. What you may or may not have done in the past does not make you less worthy. What you may or may not do in the future won't make you more worthy. Claiming your birthright of good health will give you joy and vitality and a desire to give thanks, but it will not make you more worthy. You are worthy just because God created you. This is the gift of God's grace to us, that we are accepted just as we are. Our response to God's grace, then, is to accept the fact that we are accepted, as theologian Paul Tillich observed.

This past Valentine's Day, I experienced a shining reflection of the unconditional love God showers on creation in my daughters' love for their mother. One day, my older daughters (ages ten and eight) slipped into my office, clutching a well-thumbed catalog. They had found the perfect Valentine's present for their mother—a stained-glass locket. It was beautiful and just right, they said. They were determined to get it for her. There was just one problem. It cost forty dollars. They had pooled all the money they had, every penny they had earned for weeks of babysitting their younger sisters. They had twenty dollars. With every fiber in my body, I wanted to pay for the entire locket because I was so touched by what the girls wanted to do. But the gift was theirs to give. With a lump in my throat, I took their twenty dollars and added twenty dollars for the two younger girls. My wife later told me it was the most touching and cherished gift she had ever received.

> Deep down many of us don't think we are worthy of success or "worth taking the trouble for."

The gift of health and life is offered just as fully and freely to you and me. No matter where you start, you are filled with promise and potential. You have to claim that as your birthright. Natalie Sleeth must have had this promise in mind when she wrote the opening lines of her "Hymn of Promise."

In the bulb there is a flower; in the seed, an apple tree;
in cocoons, a hidden promise: butterflies will soon be free!
In the cold and snow of winter there's a spring that waits to be,
unrevealed until its season, something God alone can see.[2]

PREPARING TO TAKE BACK YOUR HEALTH

Starting down the path of high performance health requires not only faith but planning and persistence. As you pursue your goals, first trust yourself and then commit yourself to planning and follow-through.

As you work with me through this book, you will begin to develop a whole new view of your health. I would like you to start the process by taking a clear-eyed look at where your health is, where you would like it to be, and the factors in your life that are either inhibiting you or standing as assets.

One thing you will need as you plan and work is a journal. You can keep it on paper or on your computer. Personally, I find something powerful and helpful about the transfer of my thoughts and feelings to paper in black and white as my pen moves along. I can easily flip back and forth to review and add notes. But do what works best for you. You will use your journal to record the answers to the assign-

> No matter where you start, you are filled with promise and potential. You have to claim that as your birthright.

ments I give you, to record your plans, and to keep track of your progress. You will also use it to talk to yourself—to share ideas or insights that strike you as important.

MAKING IT PERSONAL

Below is your first assignment. Take a few moments to record your answers in your journal so you can keep track of them. While the answers to these questions will undoubtedly evolve over the course of our time together, your answers will provide a preliminary glimpse of where you are now and where you could be.

1. What are your current health challenges and opportunities?
2. What are your health and life goals for the future? (Write goals for one week, one month, one year, and five years.)
3. What are your assets for achieving these health goals?
4. What are your barriers to achieving these health goals?

3 | MASTERING THE BASICS

Two roads diverged in a yellow wood,
And sorry I could not travel both
And be one traveler, long I stood
And looked down one as far as I could
To where it bent in the undergrowth.
　—ROBERT FROST, "THE ROAD NOT TAKEN"

If I had known I was going to live this long,
I would have taken better care of myself.
　—MICKEY MANTLE

When it comes to transforming your health from its current status to high performance health, what separates people who succeed from those who don't? The thousands of patients we have cared for at Rippe Health Assessment and Rippe Lifestyle Institute have taught us two important secrets. Often, these individuals came to us with their lives wildly out of control. Many were sedentary or overweight or had various health challenges or were unhappy. But they all came to us for one

31

overriding reason: they wanted to get more out of life. I would like to say all of them succeeded, but many did not.

The successful individuals tapped the power of two basic secrets. First, they mastered "the basics." I will review these basics in this chapter. Second, they made change a slow and incremental process. This mind-set actually empowers your ability to move forward.

The basics of high performance health consist of seven key strategies that anyone can adapt to personal needs and goals. In this chapter, I'll review the concepts and offer you some tips and resources. Using these strategies, you can then shape your plan for gradual, incremental change. When it comes to making positive changes for health, most people do not falter on some big cosmic issue; they falter because they don't figure out how to break up a task into small, easily achievable pieces that can fit within the context of their lives.

> The basics of high performance health consist of seven key strategies that anyone can adapt to personal needs and goals

Joan discovered the power of both of these secrets—mastering the basics and implementing them through a step-by-step plan.

MINING THE SECRETS OF SUCCESSFUL CHANGE

When Joan first came for a health evaluation, she was forty-three years old and the mother of two teenagers. In her successful career, she had risen to vice president of human resources for a Fortune 500 company. She spent her days counseling people about how they could improve their performance in the company, and she was very good at it. However, she had not been as successful, she realized, at managing her own overall "fitness," as described in the circle of values.

Over the years, Joan had slipped into a sedentary lifestyle. At first she hardly noticed any change. When she had her first child in her late twenties, she gained over fifty pounds during pregnancy but lost only thirty after the child's birth. After her second child's birth, she retained another twenty pounds. So in her mid thirties, Joan was about forty pounds heavier than she had been at age twenty. She convinced herself that a little weight gain was not too much of a problem. After all, most of her friends were also gaining weight. Her husband, Bill, seemed just as happy with her. She told herself that it was okay to be "pleasingly plump." Meanwhile, apart from her pregnancy-related weight gain, Joan added about a pound a year (like most American adults).

When Joan first arrived for her health assessment, she was about sixty pounds heavier than she had been when she graduated from college. At five foot five, she weighed 187 pounds. She knew she was overweight; a normal weight based on her body mass index would have been under 150 pounds. But she had no idea that being overweight had already begun to cause health problems. Her fasting blood sugar was 125 mg/dL; the normal range is below 100 mg/dL. Both her cholesterol and triglycerides were in the mid 200s; the healthy goal for total cholesterol is under 200 mg/dL and for triglycerides below 150 mg/dL. Her waist circumference was 38 inches, where the recommended maximum for women is 35 inches. Her blood pressure was 140/88, indicating borderline stage 1 high blood pressure; the normal range is below 120/80. Her walk on the treadmill indicated her fitness level was 10 percent below average for her age. A high-speed CT scan of her coronary arteries showed some minor areas of calcium in two of the three coronary arteries, which may be early indicators of heart disease.

Joan and I knew that she had to make some changes. We made a plan to fit her needs and schedule. She started seeing the recommended nutritionist on a weekly basis and began a regular walking program. A year later, I almost couldn't believe my eyes when I saw Joan for her annual health evaluation. She was thirty pounds lighter and looked a decade younger. She had not yet reached some goals, but her health parameters were all headed clearly in the right direction. Her blood pressure had decreased to 130/80, placing her in the "prehypertension" stage and headed toward normal. Her fasting blood sugar had fallen to 100, right at high normal. Her triglycerides were 115, and her total cholesterol was 160, within "normal" ranges but not the lower targets we had set, given her risk for heart disease. Perhaps most important, Joan viewed her life in a whole new way. She told me that she was happier and more energetic than she had been in twenty years. Plus she was looking forward to fitting into a size 8 dress the next spring for her daughter's wedding.

If this were an infomercial, I'd tell you that Joan's path was easy, but it wasn't. It's hard for almost everyone to break deeply ingrained habits. Joan had to rethink and recast both her eating and exercise patterns. She had to learn portion control and make a commitment to walk thirty minutes each day. At first she struggled, but she took the changes slowly. She learned what my colleagues at Weight Watchers call "flexible restraint" in eating and slowly cut back on the number of calories she consumed each day without depriving herself. She built up her walking program slowly, starting out at five minutes per day and progressing to thirty minutes a day over three months. At the end of the first ninety days, she felt so much better about herself that these behaviors became self-reinforcing. As a result, within one year, she was well on her way to meeting all her goals.

> If you were to take only one step to improve your health, that step should be increasing your physical activity.

Two years later, Joan had lost an additional fifteen pounds and could not imagine a day without an invigorating walk. Her fasting blood sugar, cholesterol, and triglycerides were all close to optimal. Her fitness level had climbed to 15 percent higher than average for a forty-six-year-old woman. When I asked her how she felt, she replied, "Things are so much better in my life that I am never going back. I didn't know how out of control I was until I started taking steps to win back control of my life and health." And, oh yes, she did fit into that size 8 dress for her daughter's wedding. But most important, she had dramatically reduced her risk of heart disease and diabetes and was enjoying the vitality of high performance health.

I could match Joan's success story with hundreds more. As you can see, Joan succeeded because she incorporated some basic changes in her life in an incremental way that did not turn her life upside down.

You, too, can use the same seven fundamental strategies—the "basics"—to start down the path of high performance health. They are:

1. Physical activity
2. Weight control
3. Improved nutrition
4. Improved hydration
5. Improved sleep and rest
6. Creating a positive environment for change
7. Mastering the mind-set

BASIC 1: PHYSICAL ACTIVITY

If you were to take only one step to improve your health, that step should be increasing your physical activity. Why? First, our bodies were designed to be in motion. So physical activity keeps all the body's systems tuned for health. Second, numerous medical studies have confirmed this health-promoting power of regular physical activity. Let me give you an example.

In 1995, the Centers for Disease Control and Prevention conducted an analysis of forty-three major studies that examined the relationship between physical activity and good health. When the researchers compared physically active people to inactive people, they found that the inactive people were almost twice as likely to die of heart disease compared to the active people. To put this in perspective, if you make the choice to be inactive, you have accepted the same increased risk of cardiac disease as if you smoked a pack of cigarettes per day! Now, by

CDC criteria, 60 percent of adults are truly "inactive." Unfortunately, 10 percent of adults in the U.S. still smoke a pack of cigarettes per day. Thus, in inactivity, we have a risk factor for heart disease as powerful as smoking a pack of cigarettes per day and six times as prevalent![1]

In the years since the CDC study, many additional studies have confirmed these findings and provided more evidence for the health and longevity benefits of physcal activity in specific groups of people, such as men, women, and older adults.

Despite the overwhelming evidence of the health benefits of just a moderate amount of moderate physical activity, Americans have drifted into a sedentary lifestyle. The *Surgeon General's Report on Physical Activity and Health* in the mid-1990s found that only 22 percent of the adult population in the U.S. got enough regular physical activity to result in health benefits.[2] In the years since then, as a nation we have not become any more active.

Why have we drifted into this sedentary, unhealthy lifestyle? We certainly know better. A few years ago, a *USA Today* poll asked Americans, "Do you believe that regular exercise is important for good health?" More than 95 percent of respondents gave a resounding "Yes!" So how do we explain the fact that only 22 percent of adults in the United States exercise on a regular basis?[3]

The challenge is clearly to figure out how to close the gap between what we *know* we should be doing and what we *are* doing. As my team has worked with thousands of individuals, we have concluded that the biggest barrier may be that most folks think regular activity requires a huge and strenuous effort.

This attitude reminds me of the story of a woman in the 1940s who lived deep in the Georgia countryside near the state line between Georgia and Alabama, which incidentally is also the line between the eastern and central time zones. The only traveling she did consisted of once-a-month trips into town some twenty-five miles away. But she loved the idea of travel. When the phone lines finally came to the farm, she placed a call one Saturday morning to ask a question she'd long pondered about traveling to Birmingham, a journey of about sixty miles.

"Greyhound Bus Station. May I help you?" answered the man at the other end of line.

"Yes sir," she said. "Can you tell me when the bus leaves for Birmingham?"

"One o'clock this afternoon, ma'am."

"And when does it get into Birmingham?"

"Oh, about one o'clock. Would you like a ticket?"

"No, sir. I just want to be there to see that bus take off."

When it comes to physical activity, I think most people feel they need to beat that bus to Birmingham. They think they need to train for a marathon or a triathlon or at the very least sign up for workouts and training sessions with an expensive gym membership. Nothing could be further from the truth.

During the past twenty years, my research laboratory has been the leading proponent of walking in the U.S. I also served on the CDC expert panel to recommend physical activity guidelines for Americans. The guidelines we developed made the following simple recommendation:

We urge all Americans to accumulate thirty minutes of moderate physical activity on most, if not all, days.[4]

The key words in this recommendation are *accumulate* and *moderate*. The point is that you can accumulate your physical activity in small increments throughout the day. Walk your dog in the morning. Take a brisk ten-minute walk during your lunch break. Use another ten minutes in the evening to take a pleasant walk with your spouse or children. Soon you will have thirty minutes of physical activity during the day. And the activity does not need to be intense. It should be "moderate," according to our recommendation. Thus, activities that make you out of breath are more than you need to do. What constitutes "moderate" activity? You guessed it: something like walking.

Walking, in our experience, is by far the simplest and most practical way for most people to incorporate more physical activity into their daily lives. All you need are appropriate walking shoes and comfortable, weather-appropriate clothing. Other activities that can yield multiple health benefits include cycling (either stationary or outdoor), jogging, swimming, rowing, or any other form of exercise that uses the large muscles of your body in a repetitive fashion. Even dancing qualifies. I have often thought that the *Peanuts* cartoon character Snoopy had it right when he said, "To dance is to live."

> Walking, in our experience, is by far the simplest and most practical way for most people to incorporate more physical activity into their daily lives.

Basic 1, therefore, is to find the form of physical activity that is convenient for you and work your way up to accomplishing thirty minutes of this activity on most, if not all, days. Many people like to identify two (or three) activities such as walking and cycling and alternate for variety.

In the appendix you'll find a simple walking program that starts with a short walk and progresses to thirty minutes a day. Even if you have been entirely sedentary, you can use this program.

A bonus benefit from physical activity is stress management. As a cardiologist, I know that physical activity will lower my risk of heart disease, but the major reason I *enjoy* exercising every day is that it is a great technique for stress reduction! Don't underrate this benefit of physical activity for achieving high performance health.

BASIC 2: WEIGHT CONTROL

Not surprisingly, as Americans have drifted into an increasingly sedentary lifestyle, we have also gained weight. According to the most recent statistics, more than 66 percent of adults in the U.S. are either overweight or obese.[5] Being overweight is so common in our society that we rarely notice it anymore. Ask yourself how your weight compares with your weight when you graduated from high school or college. For most adults in our country, the answer is not favorable! Because the typical adult in the U.S. gains one pound annually, individuals in their forties average twenty pounds heavier than when they were in high school or college. By the time we hit our fifties, the average gain measures over thirty pounds.

Why should you care about this? The answer is simple. Increased weight increases your risk of developing several chronic diseases. If you were a healthy weight when you were twenty years old and now are thirty pounds overweight, you have quadrupled your risk of heart disease and increased your risk of developing diabetes by between twenty and forty times what it was when you were a healthy weight. The more weight you gain, the greater the increased risk.

What are the causes of this epidemic of weight gain in our country? An enormous body of research has examined potential physical, social, psychological, and environmental contributors, but one bedrock fact lies under all these: we are eating too much and exercising too little. Sadly, not only are adults paying the price for this overindulgence, but this epidemic has also reached our children. The

> Increased weight increases your risk of developing several chronic diseases.

prevalence of obesity in children has doubled over the last twenty years. Health conditions that once occurred mainly in adulthood are increasingly appearing in children. For example, "adult onset" diabetes (type 2 diabetes) now increasingly occurs in children who are ten, eleven, or twelve years old. If we could eliminate overweight and obesity in the U.S., we could eliminate over 80 percent of all diabetes, over half of lipid (cholesterol) abnormalities, and between 40 and 70 percent of all high blood pressure. You can do your part for yourself and your family.

If you have struggled with your weight as most of us have, I don't need to tell you that losing weight and keeping it off are significant challenges, particularly since our environment offers so many high-calorie, tasty foods advertised with billions of dollars. Modern technologies have also contributed to a sedentary lifestyle in which we don't even have to get up from our couch to change TV channels. Put those calorie-packed foods together with technology that moves for us rather than keeps us moving, and we have a truly toxic environment for weight gain.

However, there is hope. There are two legitimate databases that describe the choices made by people who have lost weight and successfully kept it off. These two databases are the National Weight Control Registry and the Weight Watchers Lifetime Member Group. In order to qualify for the National Weight Control Registry (an organization some people jokingly call "the Registry of Successful Losers"), you must have lost at least thirty pounds and kept it off for at least a year. In order to qualify for the Weight Watchers Lifetime Member Group, you have to have achieved a healthy body weight and gone through a six-week program teaching you maintenance skills. The point of telling you about both of these databases is that

Good nutrition fuels your body to stay active and also helps you manage weight.

both contain thousands of individuals who have lost weight and kept it off. So while weight loss and maintenance of weight loss is hard, it is possible!

My clinic and research organization have been very active in the area of research and recommendations about weight management for many years. Recently we have partnered with Weight Watchers to perform numerous studies looking at healthy ways of losing weight. Several years ago, I wrote a book in collaboration with Weight Watchers entitled *Weight Loss That Lasts*,[6] which contains a lot of information we have developed over the years to help individuals succeed in managing weight.

Now there's no shortage of weight management and diet advice. I can reliably predict that at least one diet book annually will make the *New York Times* bestseller list. The reason there is an unending source of interest in these books is that virtually *all* of them work in the short term and virtually *none* of them work in the long term.

Based on the scientific research and our clinical experience with thousands of individuals, people who successfully lose weight invariably incorporate the following four strategies into their weight management plan.

- Regular physical activity. More than 90 percent of participants in the National Weight Control Registry exercise on a daily basis.[7]
- Sound nutrition and calorie control. This strategy doesn't mean starving or depriving yourself. Rather, it means being conscious of food choices on a daily basis, a concept that my colleagues at Weight Watchers call "flexible restraint."
- A long-term mind-set. For most of us, weight management needs to be a lifelong process rather than the self-defeating roller coaster many people get on, repetitively losing weight and gaining it back (a concept we call "yo-yo dieting").
- The support of other people. Weight management is rarely a solo act. In order to be successful at weight loss, you need the support of other people. This is what Weight Watchers achieves at their group meetings, but you can also achieve this within a supportive environment, such as your family and friends, as long as they know you are making an effort to lose weight and keep it off.

So where should you turn if your goal is weight management? I recommend Weight Watchers, which I believe is the best commercially available program using sound scientific principles to help people in the area of weight management. Weight Watchers can be found in virtually every big city and through WeightWatchers.com. Other successful programs are available, but if you are contemplating one, please make sure that it incorporates the four strategies I have described in this section.

If you are looking for a starting point for weight management, I have provided some Internet resources in the Appendix and more specific aids on our website, www.highperformancehealth.net.

BASIC 3: FUNDAMENTALS OF NUTRITION

Sound nutrition is vital to good health. Good nutrition fuels your body to stay active and also helps you manage weight. Yet most people underestimate this fact. About two decades ago, the *Surgeon General's Report on Nutrition and Health* observed that seven out of the ten leading causes of death in the U.S. have an alcohol or nutrition component.[8] In the intervening years, not much has improved. Those same seven causes still appear in the most current top twelve leading causes of death. Sound nutrition along with physical activity can help you significantly reduce your risk of such chronic diseases or conditions as heart disease, stroke, diabetes, high blood pressure, obesity, and more.

A major stumbling block in mastering the basics of sound nutrition, however, is that we suffer from almost too much information, and it's very difficult to separate the reliable information from the hype, distortion, and fantasy. Every week, for instance, popular magazines feature articles on "food for health"—some may offer balanced, evidence-based advice while others tout the latest "magical" foods, claiming health benefits well beyond what the science shows. Because news media also tend to treat the results or suggestions of single new studies as if they were absolutely true, rather than one more piece of evidence to consider in the collective light of many studies, the definition of *sound nutritional practice* often seems a moving target to consumers. So it's often hard to judge just what constitutes the basics of sound nutrition and how you can adapt those basics to your needs and tastes.

What is the best way to get started on the path of improved nutrition? I think the key is to find definitive information and put it into practice. We have to get away from the fads and the "magical" thinking that underlies many nutritional recommendations that are not based on the most recent science. Perhaps the best single source to turn to is *Dietary Guidelines for Americans,* a report developed every five years by the U.S. Departments of Health and Human Services and Agriculture and based on an extensive review of the latest scientific evidence.[9] *Dietary Guidelines for Americans 2005*, the latest version, represents a complete revision with more flexible, relevant tools for individuals. The American Heart Association and the American Dietetic Association are among the organizations that also have adopted these recommendations.

Let me summarize some of the key recommendations you'll find most useful in thinking about your nutritional practices. (You'll find the complete guidelines and other resources at www.healthierus.gov.)

- Consume a variety of nutrient-dense foods and beverages among the basic food groups. Limit intakes of saturated and trans fats (less than 10 percent of calories), cholesterol, added sugars, salt, and alcohol.
- Balance the calories you consume with the calories you burn.
- Emphasize your consumption of certain food groups. The following recommendations are based on a 2,000-calorie diet:
  - Eat 2 cups of fruit and 2½ cups of vegetables daily.
  - Choose a variety of fruits and vegetables.
  - Consume the equivalent of at least three 1-ounce servings of whole grains. Make at least half of your grain consumption whole grain.
  - Consume 3 cups per day of fat-free or low-fat milk products or calcium-rich milk product equivalents.
- Choose fiber-rich foods often. (Whole-grain breads and cereals, fresh and dried fruit, and beans and many other vegetables are fiber-rich foods.)

I selected just a few recommendations and abbreviated them, but even this list may seem a bit daunting. So here are several practical suggestions for putting them into practice in your daily life.

EAT BREAKFAST. Breakfast consumption is so important that I regard it as the most fundamental and basic rule of nutrition. My research organization has become so involved in this issue that we have teamed up with Quaker and Tropicana to establish the Breakfast Research Institute to guide professionals in the recommendation of daily breakfast consumption as one of the most powerful ways of improving nutrition available to people of all ages and stages. In fact, if you consume a healthy breakfast, you can get half of your recommended servings of whole grains and fruits each day before you take your slippers off!

SEEK THE GUIDANCE OF A PROFESSIONAL. At Rippe Health Assessment, we ask each patient to complete a three-day food record to give us a picture of his or her typical eating patterns. Then each person consults with one of our highly trained nutrition professionals to analyze current eating patterns and habits and develop a practical plan for how to use nutrition to fuel high performance health. You may find it very helpful to consult a qualified professional. The American Dietetic Association is a wonderful organization of more than sixty thousand nutritional professionals. In every major city in the U.S., you will find one or more members of the American Dietetic Association who can provide nutritional counseling for a modest fee and help you make proper food choices. To find out more about the American Dietetic Association, visit their Web site: www.eatright.org.

CONSUME MORE FRESH FRUITS, VEGETABLES, AND WHOLE GRAINS. If you emphasize just one recommendation, make it "eat more fruits and vegetables and whole grains." Chances are, you may find yourself among the 75 percent of the adult population who consume less than the recommended five daily servings of fruits and vegetables and among the greater majority who eat less than half of the whole grains recommended. If you are always on the lookout for ways that you can increase fruit and vegetable and whole-grain consumption, you will inevitably eat a healthier diet. (And, oh, by the way, you will also help control your blood pressure and your weight!)

EXPLORE SOME OF THE HELPFUL NUTRITION RESOURCES THAT SUPPORT THE DIETARY GUIDELINES. To adapt the dietary guidelines to your personal circumstances, check out the resources at www.MyPyramid.gov. This is not your old Food Guide Pyramid. Instead, it's a flexible planning tool that provides tips and resources to help you create and track your own nutrition plan. The site also has links to balanced eating plans such as the DASH Eating Plan, which was developed to help individuals lower high blood pressure but has been shown to be a flexible and enjoyable pattern for good, healthy eating for everyone.

BASIC 4: FUNDAMENTALS OF HYDRATION

I separate hydration from nutrition because hydration represents a basic, simple way of jump-starting your energy and your health. Although 25 percent of the water we consume each day comes from the solid food we eat, hydration deserves emphasis. During times of natural disaster, such as hurricanes, floods, or earthquakes, you may have observed that disaster teams first rush in fresh water, even before food. The human body can survive up to thirty days without food but no more than seventy-two hours without water. Water is a part of every biochemical reaction in our body and is essential for every aspect of life.

The human body is mostly water, in fact. Water comprises 60 percent of men's bodies and 55 percent of women's bodies. The difference in percentage derives from differences in physiology. Men typically have slightly more muscle mass, which is loaded with water; while women typically have more body fat, which contains little water.

The human body loses three quarts of water on average every day. Physically active people typically lose at least an additional quart of water. Thus, many people lose almost a gallon of water a day. When exercising or otherwise working in a warm environment, individuals can lose even more water. A typical baseball pitcher, for example, pitching a two-hour game, can lose an additional two gallons of water, as can a marathon runner, who may lose two gallons of water or more during the course of a long race. An active summer afternoon in the yard, mowing, raking, weeding, or on the tennis court will cost you plenty of extra water too. We are obligated to replace this water on a daily basis, and we do this through a variety of mechanisms, including the various beverages we drink and the foods we eat. Unfortunately, most people walk around mildly dehydrated all the time.

> Hydration represents a basic, simple way of jump-starting your energy and your health.

Why is this important? Because even mild dehydration can cause fatigue and difficulty concentrating. It can slow you down. Higher levels of dehydration can actually lead to medical problems or even medical emergencies. Most athletes and coaches now understand this and keep water or sports drinks available all the time on the sidelines of practices and games. However, the average person tends to ignore the need to drink plenty of water daily no matter his level of activity.

During the summers, I am an avid tennis player and often play for an hour with a local tennis pro. Some time ago, after a particularly grueling session on the tennis court, he confided in me that he was progressively more fatigued as each day wore on and as the summer season wore on. I gave him a simple tip: keep water on the court and stop every five to ten minutes and drink a glass of water. At our game the next week, he came to the net with a big smile on his face and told me that his problem with fatigue had entirely disappeared when he began drinking water every five to ten minutes. Furthermore, he was concentrating better than he ever had before.

The same principles apply in daily life. Years ago, I started keeping a glass or bottle of water on my desk at all times, whether I am at the clinic or in the research lab. It has made an enormous difference in terms of my ability to work long days while minimizing my fatigue. I'm happy to see more people carrying water bottles around.

One final thought about water versus other beverages: even though your body will extract water from virtually any beverage that you drink, including coffee, tea, soft drinks, or even alcoholic beverages, what the body is really calling for is pure water. If you increase your consumption of pure water, it will make an enormous difference in your energy level throughout the day. You will also benefit by not loading up your body with some of the other things contained in alternative beverages, such as sugar, caffeine, and alcohol. You have often heard the phrase "You are what you eat." There's an additional phrase that may be even truer: "You are what you drink." What your body really wants is pure water to hydrate for performance.

BASIC 5: SUFFICIENT DAILY REST

Sufficient sleep and rest are vitally important aspects of high performance health. Unfortunately, they are often neglected or underemphasized. Notice that I have separated sleep from rest. There is a great deal of overlap between the two, but they are not identical. Sleep and rest are both important to the healing and restorative processes of the body, both emotional and physical. These functions are so important that a whole section of the body's nervous system is designed to support our vital functions so that we can ignore them while we rest.

The nervous system is divided into two major divisions: the sympathetic nervous system, which fires up during times of stress and danger, and the parasympathetic nervous system, which tends to the basic housekeeping functions of the body while we are relaxing and recuperating.

> Sleep and rest are both important to the healing and restorative processes of the body, both emotional and physical.

Sometimes in medicine we refer to the actions of the sympathetic nervous system as "fight, flight, or fright" and the parasympathetic nervous system as "rest and digest." With the hustle and stress of our daily lives, we often overemphasize the "fight, flight, or fright," which can overload the body's protective defense systems without giving the equally important "rest and digest" functions time to repair the effects of that overload.

SLEEP. A recent study that followed a group of Californians for many years and tracked the key health habits that predicted good health. One of the primary factors identified as highly predictive of good health was getting seven or eight hours of sleep on a regular basis.[10] Good sleep is so important to performing at our best that it is one of the key factors that we discuss with every one of our Rippe Health Assessment patients.

Inadequate sleep is surprisingly common in our country. An estimated one out of three adults does not get adequate sleep. How is your sleep pattern? Individuals do vary, but if you get more than six and less than nine hours of sleep and do not feel sleepy during the day, your sleep patterns are probably fine. If you find that you wake up tired or get sleepy during the day, oftentimes the return to adequate sleep may be as simple as getting back on a proper routine that includes avoiding caffeinated beverages later in the evening, going to bed at a regular time, and getting involved in a regular exercise program or other way of relaxing and relieving stress. If you are overweight, snore significantly, or feel that your night's sleep is restless or intermittent, you may wish to be evaluated for sleep apnea or other sleep disorders.

A caution: I am professionally very concerned about what I view as a vast overprescription of sleep medications. Many of our patients were put on sleep medications without their primary care physician first considering personal habits that can dramatically either promote good sleep or hinder it. Public marketing campaigns for such sleep medications have subtly pushed us to think "pills" before "better practices." Before you ask for a sleep medication, try adjusting your practices.

REST. Adequate rest is just as important as sleep. Unfortunately, the technological revolution in communications, for most people, has severely curtailed the periods when we can step back from the hectic pace and stress of our daily lives and really rest and recuperate. I see the evidence all around. For many years, for instance, my family has enjoyed skiing in the beautiful mountain setting of Vail, Colorado. About

> Periods of disciplined rest are a key component of achieving balance, rehabilitation, and recuperation.

ten years ago, I noticed cell phone towers suddenly cropping up among the firs on the mountain. Soon, animated cell phone conversations babbled forth on virtually every chairlift I took up the mountain. What a shame that we were in one of the most beautiful natural landscapes in the world, yet people were so tethered to the office or other daily hassles that they couldn't even enjoy the scenery and were intruding on the enjoyment of those of us who had purposefully left our phones behind.

Now, don't get me wrong. I am a big fan of technology and am as hooked to my BlackBerry as anyone else who carries one. Nonetheless, when my family retreats to the Berkshires, I welcome the fact that my

BlackBerry goes dead and broadband Internet access has not yet arrived. Their absence helps me rest and relax in the way I intend.

Periods of disciplined rest are a key component of achieving balance, rehabilitation, and recuperation. After all, the Sabbath was designed to give us all a day of rest and meditation. Unfortunately, many of us have turned the Sabbath into another workday or a time to accomplish all the errands we didn't manage during the workweek.

I have come to understand that my daily run or swim is part of a disciplined time of rest for me. It's a time when I can get away from my other responsibilities and think about issues that may have been vexing me throughout the day. I have come to understand that these periods of exercise are crucially important to my ability to maintain balance in my life. That's why I almost always do them alone.

Disciplined periods of rest on a weekly, daily, and monthly basis are critically important to achieve the balance and perspective that are so vital to high performance health.

BASIC 6: CREATING A POSITIVE ENVIRONMENT FOR CHANGE

One key, and often neglected, aspect of change is stacking the deck in your favor by creating a positive environment for change. This is a practical consideration that makes mastering the other basics possible. The "environment" you need to manage has three facets: physical, social, and emotional.

PHYSICAL ENVIRONMENT. Creating the right physical environment for change means looking at the locales and equipment that make changing your habits easier. For example, if weight loss is one of your goals, having plenty of fresh fruits and vegetables available can be an important part of the physical environment. Make sure to put your favorite fruits and vegetables on your weekly shopping list, and keep them in an easily accessible place, such as on the kitchen counter or washed and ready in the fridge.

When it comes to physical activity, finding good walking routes or buying good walking shoes can be part of changing the physical environment to increase the likelihood that you'll carry through on your physical activity plan. I have often been astounded by patients telling me they intend to swim for physical activity, yet they don't have access to a pool or proper technique to make swimming into a key part of their permanent physical activity. As a swimmer, I know it would be impossible to swim regularly throughout the year if I did not have easy access to a local college swimming pool. One patient even told me that he was going to become more physically active with cross-country skiing. Cross-country skiing is a wonderful form of physical activity, but even in New England, we only have twenty or thirty days out of the year when cross-country skiing outdoors is even possible. Was this man going to be motivated and satisfied working the rest of the year on a ski machine? I suggested he consider adding a second activity, such as outdoor cycling, hiking, in-line skating, or walking (all good outdoor activities).

If you live in a warm climate, finding indoor places to exercise, such as a health club or even an air-conditioned mall, can be critically important in terms of increasing your likelihood of starting and sticking with an exercise program.

SOCIAL ENVIRONMENT. Having the support of your family and friends can be critically important to arriving at your goal of achieving high performance health. A supportive social environment also includes the health-care team that you will develop. A supportive social environment is so important that I have devoted the entire next chapter to building your high performance health team.

EMOTIONAL ENVIRONMENT. The third part of creating a positive environment involves internal beliefs, faith, and confidence that you can get more out of life. Your own belief system can contribute to a proper emotional environment, which is critically important and basic to starting down the path of high performance health.

BASIC 7: MASTERING THE MIND-SET

In the first chapter of this book, I challenged you to view your health in an entirely new way—not just as the passive freedom from disease but as a springboard to high performance health. In a sense, I am asking you to change your whole mind-set about health. The way you frame your health and its power to help you achieve the kind of life you want and deserve is critically important to achieving high performance health. Believing that you can have more out of life and working toward that goal are fundamental to achieving it.

While there are many aspects of mastering the mind-set, perhaps the most fundamental trait shared by all the high-performance individuals I've cared for is their ability to live in the moment. They focus on today, rather than regretting the past or fearing the future. They've mastered a concept that I call "seize the day." One person who epitomizes this is Joe Montana. During his playing days, Joe was famous for his

> The way you frame your health and its power to help you achieve the kind of life you want and deserve is critically important to achieving high performance health.

almost mystical ability to block out all distractions and remain calm while driving his team down to victory after victory in football games, including four Super Bowls. Joe epitomizes what can be accomplished when one masters the mind-set of high performance health.

You can find the techniques in your own life to live fully and completely in the present. This strategy is so important to high performance health that I will share insights into achieving it throughout this book.

CHOOSING "THE ROAD NOT TAKEN"

I started this chapter with a quote from the famous Robert Frost poem about a traveler who came to a fork in the road and had to choose one path. In a sense, I am asking you to choose your road. Often we have chosen the wrong path, the well-worn path that leads us away from the health and vitality our bodies and spirits were designed to achieve. But now you stand before two roads: one appears to be the more popular path, and the other—the road to high performance health—the less traveled. Which will you take?

Frost's traveler imagines the future "somewhere ages and ages hence" when he will be remembering the outcome of the path he is about to choose and concludes:

Two roads diverged in a wood, and I,
I took the one less traveled by
And that has made all the difference.[11]

If you choose the road to high performance health, it will make all the difference, not only in your health but in your life. We are starting on that road together, and the first step is to understand and incorporate these seven basics into your life. I am not asking you to do all of them at once but simply to be aware of these basic principles. I know they work because they are based on the experiences of thousands of high performance executives and athletes, as well as people from every walk of life who have come to our clinic and research laboratory with hopes, goals, and aspirations to achieve more in the time that God has given them on this planet. To understand the

> If you choose the road to high performance health, it will make all the difference, not only in your health but in your life.

basics and begin to incorporate them in your life is a first, but important, step.

MAKING IT PERSONAL

Your assignment for this chapter is to look at each of the seven basics of high performance health and write down one thing you can do in your daily life to incorporate or improve on that basic.

1. Physical activity
2. Weight control
3. Nutrition
4. Hydration
5. Sufficient sleep and rest
6. Creating a positive environment for change
7. Mastering the mind-set

4 | BUILD YOUR HIGH PERFORMANCE HEALTH TEAM AND ENVIRONMENT

Thank God for you,
the wind beneath my wings.

—BETTE MIDLER, "THE WIND BENEATH MY WINGS"

The happiest moments of my life have been the few which
I passed at home in the bosom of my family.

—THOMAS JEFFERSON

If you are going to master the basics of achieving high performance health, then you need to establish a true high performance health team and create an environment that supports and nourishes your high performance health goals. As I have already mentioned, most people do not falter on cosmic issues when it comes to change but on smaller, mundane issues, often related to practicality and support.

In recent years, I have enjoyed working around the country on a national hypertension education campaign with football legend Joe Montana. If you are not familiar with Joe Montana, he is perhaps the best football quarterback ever to play the game. He led the San Francisco 49ers to four Super Bowl championships in the 1980s and is the only player ever to be named Super Bowl Most Valuable Player three times. Joe was renowned for his leadership skills, particularly in the clutch—for instance, he engineered thirty-one fourth-quarter comeback wins. But in our numerous conversations, I am struck that Joe talks primarily about his team and his teammates. He often says that what made the 49ers so successful was how well they worked together and how much they trusted one another. Joe may have been the leader of the team, but his accomplishments could not have happened without the support and trust of all the men who made up that team.

> Most people do not falter on cosmic issues when it comes to change but on smaller, mundane issues.

I've never led a pro football team, but I agree with Joe's assessment of the importance of the team. I have also been blessed with phenomenal teams that work together with me at Rippe Health Assessment and Rippe Lifestyle Institute. These men and women work tireless hours and sacrifice a great deal in order to deliver the high level of caring and expertise that characterizes all we do.

You need a team too. High performance health will not occur in isolation. You need to build a team that will support and maximize your potential to help you achieve your goal of high performance health. You also need to maximize your support environment because it sets the stage for your efforts. This chapter shows you how to accomplish both of these tasks.

CAPTAINING YOUR HIGH PERFORMANCE HEALTH TEAM

Although our "high performance team" of professionals at Rippe Health Assessment at Florida Hospital Celebration Health is ready through seamless teamwork to deliver the very best care to our patients, we know that our efforts will be in vain if we don't engage patients in the belief that they can change their health. Our goal is to develop a program *together* with patients to help them achieve high performance health, but each individual must take charge of the execution, implementation, and follow-through. Each must captain his or her own team.

As captain of your high performance health team, you must start by evaluating where you are now, what matters to you most, and what supports you need to help you succeed. Before our patients arrive for their evaluations, we ask them to think about multiple aspects of their health, including a personal satisfaction inventory. I would like you to do the same. On the chart below, consider the level of satisfaction you receive from each of the individuals, groups, or factors in your life. Rate each factor individually on a scale from 1 to 5 (you aren't ranking them against each other).

> You need to build a team that will support and maximize your potential to help you achieve your goal of high performance health.

PERSONAL SATISFACTION

Example: N/A = non applicable; 1 = least satisfaction; 3 = average satisfaction, 5= most satisfaction

FAMILY	N/A	1	2	3	4	5
FRIENDS	N/A	1	2	3	4	5
SPOUSE	N/A	1	2	3	4	5
CHILDREN	N/A	1	2	3	4	5
RELIGION	N/A	1	2	3	4	5
SPORTS	N/A	1	2	3	4	5
HOBBIES	N/A	1	2	3	4	5
WORK	N/A	1	2	3	4	5
INVESTMENTS	N/A	1	2	3	4	5

COMMUNITY WORK	N/A	1	2	3	4	5
OTHER (please specify)						
_____	N/A	1	2	3	4	5
_____	N/A	1	2	3	4	5
_____	N/A	1	2	3	4	5

Have you had to make any personal sacrifices to achieve success? (Describe them briefly.)

As you can see, the personal satisfaction inventory surveys many aspects of your life, but it's not by accident that we list family, friends, spouse, and children at the top of the list. In our experience with thousands of high performance individuals, the people in those four relationships are key members of every high performance health team.

Where are your strongest satisfactions? From which people or environments do you experience the most support and enjoyment? Note your answers in your journal and keep those relationships in mind. If you are not spending enough time with those people or activities that matter most, you may want to make adjustments. In the rest of this chapter, I discuss briefly how you can build these satisfactory relationships and factors into your performance team and how you can transform areas that may present challenges.

BUILDING YOUR HIGH PERFORMANCE HEALTH TEAM

Let's get started with building your high performance health team. While there are many potential members of the team, the process starts very simply—with you.

1. YOU. To turn your health into a dynamic platform for high performance, you may first need to affirm that you are responsible for your own health. This affirmation may require a shift in thinking. But you can do it. Regardless of your circumstances or health challenges, you can take charge of your health and build a team to help you.

I can hear you saying in response, "I've looked at all those basics you want me to master—and it's clear you don't understand that I barely have time to get through each day now. And now you're asking me to add extra health practices? I don't see it." We have heard similar protests (and excuses— no time, no facility, too much travel, no interest) thousands of times at our clinic and research facility. Of course, change is hard, but I can assure you that you *do* have time. And once you see the power of turning your health into a performance tool (and, not coincidentally, see how much time high performance health frees up), you will never go back. I often remember how Bill made that discovery.

> You can take charge of your health and build a team that will help you achieve the performance and life that you want and deserve.

A high school administrator, Bill came to our research facility to participate in a walking and weight-loss research project. He was fifty-seven years old and thirty-five pounds overweight. Like many people in their fifties, he had gradually become more sedentary and watched the pounds slowly accumulate. He didn't believe he had the time or energy to do otherwise. He worked forty-five to fifty stressful hours a week at the high school, and on evenings with no meetings, he was so tired that after dinner he "chilled" in front of the television set, consuming snacks as he watched his favorite programs and rested his "weary bones."

Although Bill was physically tired, he was also tired of being tired. That's why he entered our research project. But he was a skeptical participant, a "hard sell." He did not believe that he could really change his life. He openly doubted that walking was enough exercise to make any difference. At the beginning of the study, Bill protested, "Dr. Rippe, walking is for people my parents' age, not for me. I need something that will help me lose weight and get back into shape!" Remember, Bill was in his midfifties, so his parents were probably in their eighties.

Fortunately, as an educator, Bill knew how to follow the "teacher's" instructions in spite of his personal opinion and got started. After several weeks in our walking program, he had changed his tune! He was walking forty-five minutes a day at a brisk but not uncomfortable pace. He had also adjusted what he ate,

Don't fear the hard work of change.

consuming smaller portions and more fruits and vegetables and whole grains. After the twelve weeks of the research study, Bill had lost eighteen pounds, virtually all fat. Because he consistently exercised, he had preserved his lean muscle mass, thus preserving his metabolism and making it much easier for him to continue losing weight. Perhaps most important, Bill had changed his attitude. He told me that he felt more energy and enthusiasm for life than he had for many years. Even though the study ended after twelve weeks, Bill continued the program on his own. Over the next twelve weeks, he lost another fifteen pounds.

When I saw him at our facility three months later, he pumped my hand and exclaimed, "Thank you for giving me back my life. I have so much energy now, I almost don't know what to do with myself. I find myself mowing the lawn even when it doesn't need it. My sex life is better than it has been since early in my marriage. And I have cut five strokes off my golf game by getting my gut out of the way of my swing! You shouldn't call your program the Walking and Weight Loss Study; you should call it the High-Energy, Great-Sex, Improve-Your-Golf-Game Program!" Bill had taken control of his health and discovered it could become a dynamic springboard to high energy and a better life.

Bill's story is typical. I have seen such change hundreds of times. People come into our studies thinking that what they will gain from participating is weight loss, better control of their blood pressure, lowered cholesterol, or improvement in some other measure—but to their surprise and delight, they leave with a whole new view of themselves and what they can actually achieve. What they have really learned is the power of personal engagement as the cornerstone for building high performance health. That's why we always start with "you" on the high performance health team.

It is very difficult to achieve high performance health in isolation.

So don't fear the hard work of change. I keep on my desk a quote from Marian Wright Edelman that says, "Don't be afraid of hard work or teaching your children to work. Work is dignity and caring and the foundation of a life with meaning." If you are willing to take the responsibility for your own health and willing to put in the work necessary to change your health into high performance health, you will reap the rewards of a life of purpose and meaning.

2. YOUR SPOUSE. Perhaps the most indispensable member of your high performance health team, after yourself, is your spouse. It is very difficult to achieve high performance health in isolation. It can be done, but it is much more likely to occur if you have the love and support of another person. (If you're single, a good friend can be a mainstay.)

Numerous studies have shown that isolation is particularly dangerous to your health. In fact, one study published in the *Journal of the American Medical Association* showed that individuals who lived alone following a heart attack were almost twice as likely to suffer a significant complication or die in the six months following the heart attack.[1] When we ask our patients to list their sources of satisfaction, more than 75 percent list "spouse" as their greatest source of satisfaction.

In my own life, having a loving and supportive spouse has made an enormous difference in my health. Twelve years ago, I fell in love with a beautiful woman who changed my life and health for the better. Stephanie shares in virtually everything I do, picks me up when I am feeling low, encourages me, and supports me in every aspect of my personal and professional life. She has also given me four beautiful daughters. There is no question in my mind that my wife and daughters provide the essence of meaning to my life. They are also very important to my health. They calm me down when I am too uptight and remind me that there is more to life than work. Equally important, they give me an opportunity to give love and get support in return. Having another person with whom to share both triumphs and disappointments makes an enormous difference in your ability to achieve high performance health (and in their ability too).

You may be reluctant to ask your spouse or friend to join your high performance health team. In one of our early walking studies, I remember Ruth, who told me, "It feels selfish to me to take thirty to forty-five minutes each day to go for a walk." I encouraged her to share with her husband what she hoped she would accomplish with her exercise program and perhaps even encourage him to participate. A week later she came back, smiling ear to ear, to tell me, "Joe said that if it was good for me, it was good for the family—and he even agreed to join me on my fitness walks!" Remember, the person who loves you the most wants all the best things for you, including the very best for your health. The end bonus will be that everyone who is close to you will reap benefits from your high performance health.

3. FAMILY. Every person who has been blessed with children knows that parenthood changes your life radically and wonderfully. When I first gazed into the eyes of my newborn daughter, I felt I had truly seen the face of God. I wanted to be and do my best for this wonderful new life. We always encourage patients at our research laboratory and clinic to find ways to engage their families in high performance health. Whether taking family exercise outings, finding ways to improve nutrition for every family member, or going on a restful vacation or spiritual retreat, your family can be an important source of energy to build high performance.

Just as important, while you are working on your own high performance health, you will be setting a path and standard for your children to emulate. Many studies show that a powerful predictor for children' adopting the health-promoting habit of regular physical activity is whether their parents engage in regular physical activity.[2] I know that you, like me, want what's best for your children. So

> Your family can be an important source of energy to build high performance.

don't forget that by working on your own high performance health, you can help your children understand what they can achieve with their own health and life.

4. FRIENDS. The Beatles had it right when they said, "I get by with a little help from my friends." Friends, like family, can provide support that touches and strengthens us in all aspects of our being.

Rad Smith, my college roommate, was one of my best, lifelong friends. We met our first day at Harvard, when this very tall guy ambled into our dorm suite. Rad was a phenomenal athlete (a high school All-American swimmer), and we shared an interest in poetry and academics. As we grew into and through adulthood, Rad was there for me. He was a sounding board and a support, and he never hesitated to challenge me when he felt I wasn't living up to the highest standards I had for myself or that he thought I owed myself.

Then in his early fifties, Rad was diagnosed with lung cancer, though he never smoked a cigarette in his life. He lived only six months. Such a devastating blow, such deep grief. Yet something in the refining fire of impending death helped Rad find the voice he had sought for his entire life. During those last months, he wrote some of the greatest poetry I have ever read. And he was so fully alive—and still there amazingly for his friends. I will never forget the last thing he said to my wife and me as I held his hand. He squeezed my hand, and then, looking past me to Stephanie, he said, "Never stop loving this man;

he needs you more than you will ever know." How like Rad to think about me and my needs on his deathbed. His life is still touching others through his poetry, which was published nationally after his death, and even more in the lives of his friends, like me, who cherish his friendship still, and are supported by it, inside, where the wellsprings of vitality are.

Friendship offers so many mutual benefits. There is extensive medical literature on the value of friends and community in terms of overall health benefits. One of the dangers in the frenetic pace and stress of pursuing our business and professional goals is that we often neglect our friends and don't spend the time necessary to build true friendships. What inevitably suffers is our health.

5. HEALTH-CARE PROFESSIONALS. The incredible teams of health-care professionals who care for patients at Rippe Health Assessment and guide research subjects at Rippe Lifestyle Institute include physicians, nurses, nutritionists, exercise physiologists, and pharmacists. Even if you do not have the resources of a research laboratory or clinic (and few people do), it is possible to surround yourself with a team of healthcare professionals who can help you achieve high performance health. Here are my recommendations.

Physician. The doctor-patient relationship is the cornerstone of effective medicine. But the economic model and insurance constraints operative in American medicine have taken a toll on doctor-patient relationships. Our patients at Rippe Health Assessment frequently say how wonderful it is to spend two hours over the course of a day's evaluation having in-depth discussions with a physician about health concerns and opportunities to improve health. I am

> It is possible to surround yourself with a team of health-care professionals who can help you achieve high performance health.

not suggesting that your physician needs to spend two hours with you when you come in for your annual checkup (extended health evaluations understandably have a price tag); however, you can establish and nurture an ongoing relationship with a physician who is interested in treating you as a whole person rather than a number. This may take some research on your part, but there are physicians who are willing to do this in every community in the United States.

What steps can you take to foster this type of relationship?

- **Come to the physician's office ready to outline your hopes and health considerations.** In the appendix, I provide an outline for the medical history that you can take with you, which may make this process more efficient.
- **Communicate clearly what you hope to achieve in the relationship.** I'm amazed that people seem so shy about expressing their expectations for their physician. Most people readily provide instructions for other professionals in their life, but with their physician, they are intimidated or shy. Yet most doctors welcome knowing more about their patients and will do their best to accommodate their patients' needs.
- **Change physicians if you need to.** If you feel that your physician is not willing or able to partner with you, I have a firm word of advice: get a new physician. Word of mouth in your community will lead you to the type of physician I am describing. Having a supportive partnership relationship with your primary-care physician can make a big difference in terms of achieving your goals of high performance health.

Other sources of medical information and support. Although nothing substitutes for the warmth and support that can be established in a supportive physician-patient relationship, the Internet provides many sources of sound medical advice. For example, I have been proud to serve on the Medical Advisory Board for WebMD (www.webmd.com), a great source of sound medical information. A list of helpful Web sites is included on the Recommended Resources section at the end of this book.

Nutritionist. For practical advice on your nutrition and eating practices, I strongly encourage you to consider at least a one-time consultation with a registered dietician. A skilled RD can help you sort through your own nutritional challenges and opportunities. Even though my wife and I use our extensive knowledge of nutrition to plan our family's approach to eating, we've found the resources of a trained nutrition professional very valuable on occasion. For example, when one of our children started gaining more weight than her pediatrician thought was desirable, we found that a consultation with a local registered dietician was very helpful. She helped us fine-tune some of our nutritional practices at home, identified a major culprit in high-fat, high-calorie school lunches, and encouraged our daughter's interest in organized physical activity. We followed up on these insights with concrete steps. Our daughter started taking a tasty but more nutritious lunch to school and eagerly launched into swimming lessons and then a swim team. Soon she was just the right weight for her age and body type and so proud of her achievements in the pool. Once after she did well in a 200-meter medley, her mother exclaimed, "My, you're becoming quite a swimmer!" "Mommy," she replied, "I *am* a swimmer." High performance thinking, indeed.

You can find a registered dietician in your community through the American Dietetic Association. They can be reached at www.eatright.org or 1-800-877-1600.

One word of caution: Many people who may advertise themselves as nutritionists are not actually qualified to offer nutritional advice. Many individuals who list themselves in the Yellow Pages as "nutritionists" for example, have no formal training in nutrition. If you are looking for a nutritionist, check with your physician to find out whom he or she would recommend, or look for the professional credential of "registered dietician," which certifies that the holder has earned an ADA-accredited college degree in nutrition, has completed an accredited, supervised practice program, has passed a national certification exam, and regularly engages in continuing education.

Online resources of sound nutritional information. The Internet offers a cornucopia of nutrition sites. The quality of the information ranges from excellent to misleading to worthless. Three good general sites offering evidence-based information are www.eatright.org (American Dietetic Association); www.MyPyramid.gov (tools based on *Dietary Guidelines for Americans 2005*); and www.nutrition.gov (U.S. Department of Agriculture).

Exercise physiologist. Regular physical activity is a key health-promoting behavior. You can't achieve high performance health unless you get the right amount of physical activity for you. This goal is so important that every patient leaves Rippe Health Assessment with a customized personal physical activity program, designed with the help of one of our team of exercise physiologists working under the direction of Dr. Ted Angelopoulos. Our goal is to make sure each patient's exercise program is safe and effective and fits his or her interests and environment.

Almost every community offers good resources to supply you with sound advice about how to increase physical activity in your daily life. Many local hospital wellness centers, YMCAs, or quality fitness centers have trained professionals who can guide you in this area. One resource I recommend for locating a quality health club is the trade association IHRSA—International Health, Racquet, and Sportsclub Association. Most cities have one or more IHRSA members. IHRSA clubs have a strict code of conduct and typically hire high-level professionals who are qualified to prescribe exercise and physical activity. You can locate a club using their consumer Web site, www.getactiveamerica.com.

Pharmacist. Don't forget your neighborhood pharmacist as a source of valuable information, not only about prescription medicines but also about over-the-counter medications and supplements. At Rippe Health Assessment, our team of pharmacists consults with each patient to help them understand the health purposes of their medications and appropriate uses as well as to evaluate any supplements they may be taking or considering taking. Your pharmacist will be happy to play the same role for you.

6. OTHER SUPPORTIVE PARTNERSHIPS. Beyond your family and health-care team, you have other groups of people who can guide and support you along the way.

Partners in pursuing high performance health. I always encourage people who are trying to achieve high performance health to form a partnership with someone else who has like-minded goals. Of course, this may be your spouse or significant other, but if not, then reach out and find a partner who can join you, or, even better (or in addition), find a supportive group of like-minded individuals who can help you with your goals. Such groups may be focused on one facet of your plan, such as increased physical activity, weight loss and management, smoking cessation, or improved spiritual health.

> I always encourage people who are trying to achieve high performance health to form a partnership with someone else who has like-minded goals.

Mentors. Don't be afraid to reach out to a mentor. In my life, I have been blessed to have several mentors who at critical junctures helped me see through current difficulties, discern possibilities, or get to the next stage in my life. For example, in medical school, one of my mentors was Dr. Joe Alpert, who remains a dear friend. Joe is one of the nation's outstanding clinical cardiologists. I met Joe while I was a second-year medical student at Harvard Medical School. He not only played a critical role in helping me get through med school, but he also guided me toward a career in cardiology. At every critical juncture in my professional life, he was there offering clear-sighted advice, wisdom, support, and friendship. Don't be embarrassed or shy about asking someone to be your mentor.

Spiritual adviser. A critical aspect of high performance health is understanding and employing its spiritual dimension. Numerous studies in our research laboratory and in many other settings have shown profound connections between mind, body, and spirit.

While I consider myself a very religious person, I have drawn spiritual advisers from a variety of settings, including my colleagues at Florida Hospital, who have guided me in my thinking and reading about spiritual matters. Within the past year, for example, my friend Brian Paradis guided me to the book *Wild at Heart* by John Eldredge,[3] which stimulated my thinking about the dynamic interaction of passion, desires for freedom and adventure, masculinity, and spirituality. Another spiritual adviser, Dr. Des Cummings, recommended that I read *The Return of the Prodigal Son* by Henri Nouwen,[4] which provoked profound meditation on the meaning of fatherhood and sonship.

> I strongly urge you to consider attention to spirituality and a spiritual "support community" as a key component of high performance health.

Potential spiritual advisers are all around you. It need not be a "formal" relationship. I consider myself blessed to have a variety of spiritual advisers whom I connect in various ways. I strongly urge you to consider attention to spirituality and a spiritual "support community" as a key component of high performance health.

CONSTRUCTING A HIGH PERFORMANCE HEALTH ENVIRONMENT

I hope that someday you have an opportunity to visit Rippe Health Assessment's fabulous facility located at Florida Hospital Celebration Health, outside of Orlando, Florida. I have often called the Florida

Hospital complex the Taj Mahal of American medicine because it looks more like a five-star resort than a health-care facility. Stepping into such a beautiful and inviting space gives me a lift when I head to my office. Interestingly, however, when our patients comment on their experience at Rippe Health Assessment, they seldom mention our gorgeous facility. Rather, over and over, they praise the caring environment and warm familylike atmosphere that is created both in our clinic and in our research environment. The lesson you can take from our experience is that having a wonderful facility may be a great asset, but you do not need a luxury facility in order to achieve high performance health. What you need is an environment that encourages you to be your best.

As captain of your high performance health team, you have to take responsibility for creating that environment. You can't expect your physician or your family or friends to take the lead.

Creating a positive environment that encourages and supports change includes both physical surroundings and equipment and more intangible factors. Here are some important considerations in constructing your high performance environment.

CREATE A SUPPORTIVE PHYSICAL ENVIRONMENT. Positive attributes of our physical environment provide health benefits and help shape our well-being. For example, classic studies conducted by a researcher at Yale showed that nursing home residents who cared for a pet or tended plants derived multiple health benefits from these simple practices. These people were less likely to get infections, had better control of their blood pressure, and in general lived longer than individuals who did not have this type of opportunity to interact with their environment. Other studies show

> You do not need a luxury facility in order to achieve high performance health. What you need is an environment that encourages you to be your best.

benefits from living with pets or gardening or just getting out regularly into nature.[5]

I have personally experienced the value of creating a positive environment to promote my health. I work in a large, airy study filled with blooming orchids. Near my desk is a living coral reef tank, and classical music is always playing softly in the background when I am at work. I know that these aspects of my environment allow me to work at the high level I expect of myself.

Here are some suggestions for setting up your physical environment to enhance your mastering three of the high performance health "basics" discussed in Chapter 3.

1. **For physical activity.** Make sure your environment includes mapped-out walking trails or routes of various distances. Identify inclement weather alternatives if your main activity takes place outdoors. Purchase good equipment for whatever physical activity you choose—if you're going to walk, that means good walking shoes and weather-appropriate, nonbinding clothing. Arrange times and places to meet other people to participate with you.

2. **For nutrition.** Make sure your pantry, refrigerator, and freezer are stocked with healthy foods and that you always have at least two or three different choices of fresh fruits available for easy snacking. Make a list before grocery shopping to help you stick to your new choices and avoid temptations.

3. **For weight management.** Make sure you've planned for physical activity and that you have healthy foods available. Clear out the pantry of calorie-empty snacks and drinks, if possible. Create a positive environment with supportive individuals. Don't let yourself get too hungry between meals. Consider joining a support group, such as Weight Watchers, to assist in your efforts.

You get the point: taking simple steps to tilt the environment in your favor is very important, particularly as you begin the path to high performance health.

Find a third place. Years ago, when he was editor of *American Health Magazine*, my friend T. George Harris alerted me to an emerging body of literature that identified the importance of "a third place" for everyone seeking improved health. The growing research supported the idea that most people who were able to improve their health had discovered an important "third place" in their lives, beyond home and work. At such third places, we are typically surrounded by caring individuals who share like interests or missions and who support not only who we currently are but who we hope to be. For many people, this third place is their church or faith community. For others, it may be a health club, social or fraternal club, garden club, volunteer group, book club, hobby group, or the like. The point is that finding another place where you can be connected yields multiple health benefits.

> **Most people who were able to improve their health had discovered an important "third place" in their lives, beyond home and work.**

Volunteer. Would it surprise you to hear that one of the best things you can do for yourself is to do good for others? Numerous studies have shown that individuals who volunteer for worthy causes that help others, derive multiple health benefits for themselves. For example, a study that has followed more than eight thousand people in California for twenty-five years has identified seven factors that lower the risk of chronic disease and improve longevity.[6] One of the key factors is participation in regular volunteer work. Isn't it wonderful to know that the unselfish act of doing good for others also yields important benefits for our own health?

Why do volunteers typically experience better health? No one knows for sure, but the theories point toward the important physical and spiritual health benefits of being connected to each other.

CREATE A POSITIVE MENTAL ENVIRONMENT. So far in this section, we have focused on various external aspects of constructing a high performance environment. There is an equally important aspect that deals with your "internal" environment. Have you created a mind-set for high performance health? Are you willing to truly take the next step toward turning your health into a performance springboard rather than a passive aspect of your life? Are you willing to connect with other people? Are you prepared to forgive other people who have hurt you? Have you forgiven yourself and affirmed that you are worthy? Are you prepared to voyage forward, not look backward? All of these issues are so important that I devote two chapters to performance thinking and the vital role of positive emotions in high performance health.

SETTING THE STAGE FOR SUCCESS

In many ways, this entire chapter has been about setting the stage to achieve high performance health. One aspect of stage setting is surrounding yourself with people who support your change, and the other aspect is building an environment that encourages and supports that change. But in the final analysis, the key factor is you. Are you ready to take those steps in your life to create not only a high performance team but also a high performance environment? If you are, you are well on your way toward success.

> The key factor is you. Are you ready to take those steps in your life to create not only a high performance team but also a high performance environment?

MAKING IT PERSONAL

Your assignment for this chapter is to identify three people whom you want on your high performance team and three changes in your environment that you are going to create to promote your high performance goals. List those people and those changes below:

Three people whom I am going to ask to join my high performance health team and what I am going to ask them to do:

    1. _____

    2. _____

    3. _____

Three changes I am going to make in my environment to turn it into a high performance environment:

    1. _____

    2. _____

    3. _____

5 | TRANSFORM YOUR LIFE THROUGH HIGH PERFORMANCE THINKING

We are what we repeatedly do. Excellence, then, is not an act, but a habit.

    —ARISTOTLE, *NICOMACHEAN ETHICS*

I think it is an immutable law in business that words are words,
explanations are explanations, promises are promises—
but only performance is reality. Performance alone is the best measure of
your confidence, competence and courage. Only performance gives you
the freedom to grow as yourself.

    —HAROLD GENEEN, FORMER CHAIRMAN, ITT

Improving performance is a powerful desire for most people. What tasks do you care passionately about performing well? Where do you yearn to improve or already strive to improve? The answers usually depend on your current circumstances.

For the individual struggling to lose weight, enhanced performance may mean figuring out how to incorporate healthy eating habits or more physical activity into his or her daily life. For the individual who has had a heart attack, it may mean starting a walking program or changing some of the bad habits that may have contributed to the development of heart disease. For the individual battling cancer, it may mean keeping a positive mind-set or simply doing better the next day than the day before. For working parents, better performance may mean making more time to eat dinner regularly with their children. For the elite athlete, increased performance may mean shaving a few hundredths of a second off their best time for a hundred-meter sprint or cutting a stroke

Using your mind-set and mental attitude to frame issues positively is high performance thinking.

or two off the average round of golf. For the high-level executive, it may mean squeezing an extra fifteen minutes out of an already packed day to accomplish another business goal.

All of these people share the goal of improved performance. Yet too often they may ignore two of the most powerful tools available to them—using their health as a performance tool and their minds as a powerful ally to frame issues in their lives in a more positive and achievable light. Using your mind-set and mental attitude to frame issues positively is high performance thinking. International ski champion Diana Golden used high performance thinking to the max.

I met Diana some years ago when we were each honored to receive one of the ten annual Healthy American Fitness Leaders Awards from the President's Council on Physical Fitness and Sports. Diana was a phenomenal athlete. The most amazing thing was that she skied on one leg. Diana had lost a leg to childhood cancer at the age of twelve but was determined to live her life fully and without regret. She trained herself to ski at the very highest levels on one leg and for eight years dominated the World and U.S. Disabled Ski Championships, winning multiple golds in every championship. What I remember most about Diana was her infectious laugh and her encouragement to others to "overcome your fears, pursue your dreams and to never give up." When the awards ceremony arrived, there was some concern that Diana might have difficulty mounting the stage to accept her President's Council accolade. "No problem!" she laughed, swinging aside her crutches and hopping up the stairs on one leg. Diana inspired us all by showing us what discipline, hard work, and the human spirit are able to accomplish. Her high performance life is also an inspiration to every person who faces a physical or medical challenge. Her

> **The essentials of high performance thinking can help you achieve your dreams.**

pure joy in being alive made everyone around her feel like a better human being. When at age thirty-eight Diana Golden died of breast cancer, the headline for her obituary captured something of her can-do spirit: "Diana Golden Wins Her Last Race, Leaves Cancer Behind."

You can accomplish whatever you can dream. The essentials of high performance thinking can help you achieve your dreams.

THE ESSENTIALS OF HIGH PERFORMANCE THINKING

What do I mean by performance? It is simply the ability to do those things in your daily life that are fulfilling and bring you meaning and happiness. It's the ability to meet the challenges that life flings at you without losing your equilibrium or core confidence. It's the ability to keep moving toward your goals, whether the way is smooth and beautiful or stormy and rough.

The key quality that distinguishes people who are able to perform—whether they are news-making elite athletes or executives or the unsung heroes of "regular America"—is their ability to employ high performance thinking. High performance thinking in all its aspects draws on the powerful connections between our minds, bodies, and spirits. In this chapter, I look at how you can tap this vital connection between mind, body, and spirit through eight aspects of high performance thinking. These eight traits can enable you to transform your mind-set into a powerful ally for high performance health and high performance living.

1. Passion
2. Trust
3. Courage
4. Discipline
5. Focus
6. Consistency
7. Happiness
8. Prayer

THE FOUNDATION OF MIND-BODY-SPIRIT CONNECTIONS

Over many years as a physician, I have seen numerous instances in which, given their medical conditions, patients defy the prognostic odds by improving or surviving.

For example, I'll never forget George, who had survived quintuple bypass surgery (despite his heart functioning at just 20 percent efficiency) only to have appendicitis strike soon after his heart surgery. As they wheeled him into the operating room to fix his acute appendicitis, the attending surgeon gravely told me he doubted that George would survive. As George rolled by, however, he winked at me and said, "Don't give away my bed, Doc." We didn't. George made it, defying the odds. Vicky, another patient, survived a complex and tumultuous three weeks in the intensive care unit with heart failure and sepsis, largely, in my opinion, because she never gave up hope.

At first, I thought examples like these were just a matter of luck, but as I matured as a physician, it became apparent to me that patients

> High performance thinking in all its aspects draws on the powerful connections between our minds, bodies, and spirits.

could dramatically change the odds in their favor by tapping into the power of their mind-body-spirit connections.

High performance athletes have long tapped into these powerful connections. Many athletes, such as golf great Jack Nicklaus, soccer marvel Pelé, Olympic champion Jackie Joyner-Kersee, or basketball legend Larry Bird, have described those transcendent moments when, completely relaxed and calm but sharply focused, they were able to perform spectacular sporting feats. Often athletes describe this special state as playing "in the zone." Jack Nicklaus captured this experience beautifully in his classic book *Golf My Way*:

> I never hit a shot, even in practice, without having a very sharp, in-focus picture in my head. It's like a color movie. First I "see" the ball where I want it to finish, nice and white and sitting up high on the bright green grass. Then the scene quickly changes and I "see" the ball going there—its path, trajectory and shape, even its behavior on landing. Then there is a sort of fadeout and the next scene shows me making the kind of swing that will turn the previous images into reality.[1]

What Jack Nicklaus is describing is a highly disciplined, elite athlete taking advantage of the powerful connections between mind and body. Runners and other recreational athletes often experience something similar as the emotional benefit of their physical activity. Runners often call it "runner's high." In the thousands of runs I have taken, I can't recall a single time when I haven't felt mentally and emotionally better at the end of the run.

Walking offers its highs too. For example, in a study we performed to examine the potential emotional benefits of walking on a treadmill, study participants walked for forty minutes in four different conditions: fast walking, moderate walking, slow walking, and walking at a self-selected speed. A fifth control group did not walk at all. The participants took a battery of psychological tests before and after their exercise session, then returned to their normal work environment. We paged them every thirty minutes for the next two hours and had them repeat the psychological tests. The results were astounding. No matter what speed people walked, they achieved immediate and significant psychological benefits, and the benefits lasted for the whole period monitored. I would also note that these emotional benefits came from an indoor treadmill walk, not outdoors where natural surroundings might be expected to give a boost.

Because the evidence suggests that mind-body connections are fundamental to achieving high performance health, we counsel every patient on the essentials of this resource. Understandably, some patients initially object to the idea that we are going to explore mind-body connections as part of their annual health evaluation. It doesn't take long, however, for most people to realize that we are encouraging them down a path that holds enormous power to benefit their lives. The same will happen to you if you allow yourself to tap into all of the essentials and resources of high performance thinking.

PASSION. Passion is the fuel that drives performance. At Rippe Lifestyle Institute, our motto is Passion, Commitment, Performance. We chose this motto for a very specific reason. Our research sponsors want us to bring great energy to the scientific work that we do. But passion implies more than just energy. It also implies a deep set of values and caring about a topic. These are the traits that I expect, teach, and demand of my employees and of myself. Passion is what allows people to go beyond the expected norms and accomplish incredible results in their work.

I also believe that passion is the fuel that allows some people to get more out of life than others. Passion is also the leaven that makes all the other essentials of high performance thinking rise to greater effectiveness. There's something about people with passion for life that attracts us.

Molly Yeaton walked into my life, literally, when at age seventy-five she signed up to participate in one of our research projects. Retired from forty years as a physical fitness instructor at the local YMCA, she remained passionate about her daily walking program. She attributed her vitality and good health to it. I'll say—she blew the stats for her age group off the chart. She urged others to follow her example and recruited vigorously for our walking studies. When I was ready to write the book *Fitness Walking for Women*, I knew who I wanted on the cover and in the book with coauthor Anne Kashiwa and me.

Grandma Toney, as my daughters call her, cares passionately about children and education. A strong black woman who escaped a very difficult childhood in the South, she had married and raised five children in Boston. Her career was cleaning people's houses with pride, dignity, and purpose—but her *calling* was caring and helping others achieve their best. She led by example and lavished love. Her five children all went to college, something she had

> **Passion is the fuel that allows some people to get more out of life than others.**

not been able to do. I realize now that after my mother died, Mrs. Toney took me under her wing as I finished medical school and for many years afterward. Her standards were high. "Don't mess with Mrs. Toney!" I often said. But as a person and maturing physician, I benefited from her expectation, example, and love. Now my whole family does, though Grandma Toney has been retired for some time.

In a different vein, I remember two CEOs who came for health evaluations. Their high-pressure careers meant they needed to perform at the top of their game. They didn't know each other, but they offered the same unusual chief complaint. And what "complaint" was that? Both had played high-level college basketball, but now in their fifties, neither one could dunk a basketball any longer. Both of these CEOs used their physical fitness and discipline as performance tools to accomplish their demanding jobs. Each rigorously followed an exercise program, even if it meant getting up way before dawn. They loved their lives. But that soaring ability to dunk had slipped away. Setting a dunk as a goal was, I think, a way they showed their passion for high performance living. In addition to their excellent nutrition and aerobic programs, we added some strength training. When I saw them the next year, each still derived great joy from high performance health and praised the added benefits of strength training. But could either of these fifty somethings now "slam the rock"?

> If you are passionate about your health, you will be passionate about your life—and suddenly you will start seeing good things happen everywhere.

Nope. One did proudly report that he could grab the basketball rim with both hands for the first time since his twenties. But in my book, both could "soar with the eagles."

As you think about your own road to high performance health, consider those things you are either currently passionate about or feel you could be passionate about. Those are the things that will lead you to the deep reservoir of natural energy that each of us possesses. One of my goals is to make you passionate about your health. If you are passionate about your health, you will be passionate about your life—and suddenly you will start seeing good things happen everywhere.

TRUST. Trust is fundamental to both high performance thinking and high performance health. Dr. Redford Williams has written beautifully on this topic in his book *The Trusting Heart,* in which he describes trust as the most important and effective antidote to the anger and hostility that contribute to developing heart disease. For me, trust is the attribute that allows you to let go of guilt and live for today, staying "in the moment." My colleague Dr. Monica Reed has also written insightfully about trust in her book *The Creation Health Breakthrough: Eight Essentials to Revolutionize Your Health Physically, Mentally and Spiritually,* in which she emphasizes trust as the *T* in her health-promoting acronym CREATION.[2]

Trust has three equally important components:

- Trust in yourself
- Trust in others
- Trust in God

Trust in yourself. The ability to transform your health into a powerful performance tool really starts with developing the belief that you are capable of making changes. I know it can be done. Over and over again, my team and I have seen individuals slowly develop the belief that they can change their lives forever and for the better. For many, this growing conviction starts with accomplishing small steps. Someone who has been sedentary takes a five-minute daily walk without skipping or stopping. Someone who is overweight loses the first three pounds as planned slowly over three weeks by making simple, doable modifications. Believing you can accomplish a goal is fundamental to accomplishing that goal. The good news is that trusting yourself becomes a self-reinforcing behavior, and soon you not only trust yourself in health matters but in many other aspects of your life.

Trust in others. Trust in each other is fundamental to learning and improving. As children we are able to grow, to spread our wings for first flight, and when we crash-land, to get up and try again because we trust that our parents love us, want the best for us, and will take care of us. Trust keeps us bound in love even when such childhood development results in tears or hard facts learned. As adults, we can make lasting, loving marriages and friendships only if trust is the bedrock foundation. Even my big, rambunctious Labrador retrievers are able to become cooperative, trustworthy family members because from my caring, consistent behavior toward them, they sense they can trust me and the training I give them. Being trustworthy in relationships your-

> Trust in each other is fundamental to learning and improving.

self and trusting in others to provide the same support frees you up not only to fly but to let go of certain worries.

Trust in God. Trust in God is also essential to feeling that there is order and consistency in the world. Rick Warren in *The Purpose Driven Life* writes about the importance of trusting that God has a purpose in life for each of us. I think, too, of the millions of people who have found reassurance in the Twenty-third Psalm, "The LORD is my shepherd; I shall not want . . . " (NKJV). Even in the face of trials and death, comes the promise: we shall not want. Whatever there is will be enough. There will be a way through. That way may require us to keep working hard when we can't see how anything will work out, but there will be a way. This faith in God's love echoes through the centuries in the simple but powerful statement of Julian of Norwich: "All shall be well, and all shall be well, and all manner of things shall be well."

The trust that God the Creator is ever present and ever creating within us and throughout the universe enables us to live in the moment, to seize the day. My patients who place their trust in God are invariably more able to rid themselves of anxiety and focus on the key tasks at hand to achieve high performance health and more meaningful living.

COURAGE. Change takes courage. This may not be the in-the-face-of-danger brand of courage that military personnel and rescue workers regularly summon, but it still takes real courage to look carefully at your own life and to assess both your strengths and your weaknesses as you think about ways you can improve your life and health. Often, people achieve less than they could because they draw back from looking inside their hearts for fear of what they might find. Remember you are worthy; nothing you discover by self-examination can change that. And taking small, honest steps to evaluate both where you are now and where you want to be becomes very powerful, self-reinforcing behavior. As my friend Joan Lunden, the former host of *Good Morning*

America, once said to me, "Courage is like a muscle; the more you use it, the stronger it becomes."

Stephanie demonstrated the courage to tackle a personal challenge when, after the birth of our last child, she determined to find a sport she could really *enjoy* lifelong. Until this point and through four pregnancies, she had walked and used some yoga and light strength training to bolster cardiovascular fitness and emotional well-being. But duty as much as enjoyment probably motivated her commitment. So I was surprised when she declared her intention of finding a sport. Swimming appealed to her most, and she wanted to excel, not just paddle around the pool. She found a local college coach for instruction. She found time to swim daily while caring for four daughters and a busy schedule. She ignored raised eyebrows about her desire to excel. In short order, she became a terrific swimmer. She was the first person I ever knew to master the butterfly stroke as an adult—her skill inspired me to risk trying. Because she had the courage to try something new, she found the true joy of a disciplined program of fitness that was right for her and unlocked potential she didn't know she had.

What would you like to try? Give yourself credit. It takes courage to go out and walk five or ten minutes if you have been totally sedentary. It takes courage to tell your friends that your goal is to lose twenty pounds over the next year, particularly if you have had problems losing weight and keeping it off in the past. It takes courage to ask your family to support you with your desire to stop smoking cigarettes, particularly if you have tried and failed in the past. But the good news is, if you break each of these goals into small steps and give yourself credit for having the courage to try to make change, change can and will happen.

DISCIPLINE. Most of us spend our lives trying to keep chaos at bay. It's what Henry David Thoreau meant when he wrote, "Most men live lives of quiet desperation." Every high performance individual I've ever met has developed a keen sense of discipline. This doesn't mean that they are depriving themselves of pleasure or enjoyment in life. Quite the contrary. Appropriate structure enables them to make forward progress every day. Discipline frees up space, time, and resources—not just for work on goals but for other important activities, people, and interests you value.

My wife, Stephanie, once unknowingly offered me a powerful and moving example. One night not too long before we were married, we were fixing dinner at her apartment. Lying on the kitchen table was a ledger. Seeing me glance at it, Stephanie said I could take a look. It was her financial journal. Now, you may think that full-time television anchors in major markets like Boston make major salaries—but they don't. Plus the cost of living in Boston is very high. I knew that Stephanie managed her resources with discipline in that environment, but I didn't know how scrupulously she was keeping track. The ledger recorded every paycheck and then every last expense. She had it down to the penny! Then I glimpsed something of the real heart and purpose of her accounting: every week she allowed two or three dollars to buy a couple of flowers at the local grocery store. I knew that I had fallen in love with a woman who not only had the discipline to manage her finances and her life, but also used that discipline to bring beauty into her life and placed a high value on doing so.

> Every high performance individual I've ever met has developed a keen sense of discipline.

Discipline and structure ensure that you move in a positive direction every day. They enable you to make time for *who* and *what* are most important to you. This is the reason I've asked you to keep a journal and write down your key assessments, your plans, your daily progress, and your reflections. I also encourage you to "make an appointment" in your daily planner for your exercise session. I write down every day the time when I intend to exercise. I know my workout is important to my ability to work and relieve my stress, so I don't leave it to chance to get in my forty-five-minute exercise session. You'll be surprised at how effectively this simple technique helps you consistently accomplish this important goal. I encourage you to find the structure and discipline that works for you.

FOCUS. I have known many people who are highly disciplined, but fewer who are tightly focused. During my academic career at Harvard, for example, I was surrounded by disciplined people, but many of these people were not able to focus on the key tasks or objectives they needed to accomplish each day. As a result, they didn't get the full benefit from their discipline or from all the rich educational opportunities present in the university environment.

Focus describes the ability to order tasks into priorities and devote single-minded attention to each task in order of its prioritized importance. Focus helps you conquer the many mundane distractions whose threat to performance you tend to ignore. For instance, probably like many of you, I carry a Black-Berry. However, I make it a point to answer e-mails only at certain set times. Otherwise, I can be pulled off the tasks that I need to accomplish to respond to other people's priorities. Focus turns the light of discipline into the laser of achievement.

> Focus turns the light of discipline into the laser of achievement.

CONSISTENCY. People often excuse their erratic efforts at change by misquoting the nineteenth-century American sage Ralph Waldo Emerson. "Consistency is the hobgoblin of little minds," they intone. What Emerson actually said was, "A *foolish* consistency is the hobgoblin of little minds" (my emphasis).

Continuing to treat health as the passive absence of disease is a foolish consistency. But aiming every day toward your best health now is a wise consistency. And a wise consistency is vital to accomplishing every important goal. Joe Montana emphasizes that idea with a story about his number one receiver, Jerry Rice, arguably the best pass receiver ever to play football. When Jerry Rice was a rookie, Joe said, the first time

Jerry caught a pass in practice, he ran ninety yards to the opposite end zone. All the veterans stood around laughing, thinking the clueless rookie was trying to impress the coaches. Not so, Joe said. For the rest of the fourteen or fifteen years he and Jerry Rice played together, Joe knew that in practice he could count on Jerry running the ball into the end zone every time he touched it. When Jerry Rice was asked why he did this, Joe said that he explained that his job was to catch the football and turn it into touchdowns and if he didn't go to the endzone in practice then maybe there would be a time in the game where he'd give up before reaching his ultimate goal—to score a touchdown.

You don't have to be a pro football player to reap the benefits of consistency. Taking simple steps that fit within the fabric of your day, such as finding time to consistently walk twenty to thirty minutes on most, if not all, days, or consistently paying attention to better nutrition, is the key to reaping long-term health benefits. Consistency is also the key to turning your health into a springboard for high achievement.

Routines are a fundamental way to achieve consistency in your life. I learned that lesson early. For a time as an undergraduate student, I volunteered at a halfway house for former mental patients. One day, my young colleagues and I decided to shake up the house's routine by rearranging the furniture and changing the mealtimes. We thought this would be a good way of rousting the residents out of their lethargy and maybe introducing some new patterns of thinking.

When I shared our "brilliant" idea with my faculty adviser, the eminent psychologist Dr. Robert W. White, he gently chided me to think again about how far I disrupted people's routines. "After all," he cautioned, "routines are comforting." This halfway house in particular relied on routine to provide stability and balance for its residents. Certain routines can help you focus on what is important by taking away the need to devote extra energy to things that should be, after all, routine. As an eighteen-year-old, I wasn't quite convinced, but now I'm a believer. Without routines, right down to the three-by-five cards on which I keep each day's to-do list, I could neither achieve the consistency essential to more important work nor preserve precious family time.

Recording in your daily journal what works and doesn't work for you and using that information to help you craft your own routines will lead to consistency and ultimately to higher performance for you.

If you have any doubt about the power of the right routines to produce consistency, consider the example of my friend Nolan Ryan, the Hall of Fame baseball pitcher. We met when we developed a fitness campaign for individuals over the age of forty. Nolan Ryan was a stickler for routine. He threw more no-hitters (seven) and struck out more batters (5,714) than any other pitcher ever to play baseball. He credited routine for his success. After every game, he spent thirty to forty-five minutes on a stationary cycle and then began a three- to four-day conditioning routine getting ready for his next pitching start. At the age of forty-six, in retirement, Nolan could still throw a baseball almost 100 mph—and hit his target. Many successful younger pitchers have adopted Nolan's commitment to routines for consistency.

HAPPINESS. Many of us spend considerable energy trying to figure out what will make us happy. That's a worthwhile goal, because finding true joy is essential to good health. But sometimes we may chase happiness down unreliable paths, using all the wrong "equipment."

A few years ago, one of my colleagues at our clinic recommended a book by Richard Leider and David Shapiro called *Repacking Your Bags*. This friend was concerned that I was so busy pursuing both career and better health-care causes that I was not leaving enough room in my life to find true happiness. "Read it!" he said.

The book's fundamental concept springs from a pivotal question that a native guide asked Richard Leider while he was leading a trek for midlife adventurers through the Serengeti Plains in East Africa. On one day's trek through a particularly beautiful area, the guide kept eyeing the high-tech backpack Leider was carrying. It was "covered with snaps, clasps, and zippers, full of pockets and pouches, compartments inside compartments, a veritable Velcro heaven—and I have the thing stuffed," writes Leider. With the pack, he was prepared for anything that might happen to his group. In contrast, the guide carried a single spear. At the end of the trek, Leider offered to show the pack's contents and features to the guide, who had seemed fascinated by it. Proudly, Leider spread out all the stuff—hundreds of items, it seems. The guide looked at the array, silent but seemingly amused, and then asked, "Does all this make you happy?"[3]

Many of us spend considerable energy trying to figure out what will make us happy.

The question catapulted Richard Leider into a period of deep reflection. One result was the book *Repacking Your Bags*, in which the authors provide an excellent guide to focusing on those issues that bring you joy while jettisoning distractions that keep you from that goal.

I struggle to take my own medicine, I must admit. I continue to struggle to balance the demands of a busy professional life with my family and their needs. I can't say that I have my "bags" packed exactly right just yet, but I know one thing for certain: those things which bring me joy also bring me good health, and such joy and happiness are essential to good health.

PRAYER. Prayer is empowering. It's also individual. For me prayer is many things. It is opening oneself to communication with God—a wordless sense of living in God's presence. Prayer is listening. It is, as the poet wrote, "the soul's sincere desire, unuttered or expressed."[4] And it is also an intentional speaking and sharing of our deepest concerns and hopes and promises.

When my wife and I decided to have a family, we were both somewhat older than the optimum age to do this: I was forty-eight, and she was thirty-seven. As we sought to get pregnant, each time we began the process with a prayer asking God not for a specific outcome but for guidance and for the wisdom to follow His path. We promised in return that if we were blessed with a child, we would do our very best to be devoted parents. We have subsequently been blessed with four beautiful children who have filled our lives with joy and meaning beyond what I could have imagined. I tell you this story not because our prayers were answered, but because both of us felt the need to pray.

The need to engage in prayer is extremely common when we face big issues, uncertainties, or dangers. One study published several years ago, for example, documented that more than 95 percent of patients facing open-heart surgery prayed the night before.[5] I have often thought that we in medicine are missing an enormous opportunity to help our patients by not offering to pray with them. Fortunately, I believe this is beginning to change.

> I encourage you to explore prayer as a way of enhancing high performance thinking.

I view the main benefit of prayer as an organizing principle and source of comfort that links each individual to a sense of a larger mission and order in the universe controlled and watched over by the Creator. I encourage you to explore prayer as a way of enhancing high performance thinking.

THE PATHWAY TO PERFORMANCE THINKING

In his insightful book *Mind as Healer, Mind as Slayer*, Dr. Ken Pelletier reminds us that the mind can be both a powerful force for healing and a negative force that plays tricks on us, ultimately becoming a "slayer."[6] This chapter has focused on those aspects of performance thinking that tap the power of the "mind as healer." In the next, we will focus on how to overcome negative emotions that, left unchecked, can turn the mind into a "slayer."

For now, I want to leave you with the hope and understanding that you can tap into the phenomenally powerful connections between mind, body, and spirit through the eight components of high performance thinking outlined in this chapter. Your next step is to start to work on that goal.

MAKING IT PERSONAL

To start focusing on performance thinking, think about the following:

List three ways that you are going to work on improving the level of trust in your life:

1. _____
2. _____
3. _____

List three ways that you are going to establish positive routines in your daily life:

1. _____
2. _____
3. _____

List three aspects of your life in which you find true happiness and ways that you will work to increase that level of happiness:

1. _____
2. _____
3. _____

6 | REVITALIZE YOUR HEALTH THROUGH EMOTIONAL WELL-BEING

Huffy Henry hid the day,
Unappeasable Henry sulked.
I see his point,—a trying to put things over.
It was the thought that they thought
they could do it made Henry wicked & away.
But he should have come out and talked.

    —JOHN BERRYMAN, *THE DREAM SONGS,* #1

So faith,
hope,
love abide,
these three;
but the greatest of these is love.

    —1 CORINTHIANS 13:13

Far too many books about health speak only about physical health and neglect emotional well-being. As I have grown older (and I hope wiser), I have come to believe that to ignore the vital emotional aspect of our lives is a terrible mistake when it comes to our health. After all, we are not merely physical beings with no mental life, nor are we simply spirits with no physical being. We are both. Each of us is a complex being with an exuberant emotional life inextricably woven together with a complex physical existence. We ignore the interconnections between our emotions and our bodies at our peril.

I would go a step further: if we do not examine and understand how to channel, control, and modify our emotions, it is very unlikely that we will achieve high performance health. Unlike Berryman's Henry, you and I must not huff and "hide the day"; no matter what our reactions to the multiple forces that impinge on our lives and feelings, we must "come out and talk." We may not be able to control many of those external forces and the stress they generate, but we can "talk" with ourselves, look within, understand our emotional responses and reactions, and examine how some may block health and well-being and how others may support and nourish health.

This chapter focuses on several major emotions that are key to achieving your best health now, on the triggers for these emotions, and on the potential emotion-driven behaviors that can either present challenges that can kill your efforts to achieve high performance health or offer wonderful opportunities to use emotional and mental strengths as life-giving "healers" on the path to high performance health.

WHO'S IN CONTROL? WHAT'S IN CONTROL?

Why do some people always seem centered and in control of their lives no matter how tough their circumstances, while other people seem flattened by the most minor of difficulties? One answer may lie in the psychological concepts of "internal locus of control" versus "external locus of control." People who have an "internal" locus of control believe that their own habits and actions and the way they approach the world have an enormous impact on their health and their lives. They believe that this control resides within themselves. In contrast, people who have an "external" locus of control tend to believe that their lives are controlled by external forces that are largely beyond their power to influence.

The possibility of achieving your best health now grows from an internal locus of control—your belief that you can do it or, at least, your belief that you can take the first steps and go from there. You have an enormous opportunity to control your health and your path in life. Doing so requires turning your emotional life into a powerful ally. We're going to explore how to do that in this chapter.

Many years ago, I had a sudden insight into how powerfully one's emotional perspective can frame reality and drive behavior. I was an avid student of karate. Fixated on the goal of a black belt, I worked out in the karate studio several hours a day. After a year's study, I'd advanced well up the ranks, but "experienced" doesn't mean "perfect." During one fast-moving exercise, I inadvertently kicked another student—hard! Fortunately, the other guy was okay, but I broke a big toe. Now, if you've ever broken a toe, you know it can really hurt. And each step sharply reminds you of just how much. Then and now, medical treatment for broken

> The possibility of achieving your best health now grows from an internal locus of control.

toes is limited; neither casts, splints, nor "boots" work, so we doctors basically advise patients to stay off their feet as much as possible and let the bone heal. Well, I was not about to do this: after a week of hobbling on crutches, I discarded them and resumed walking around and also exercising in karate. But I took consolation in complaining bitterly and, I fear, constantly about how much it hurt. After putting up with this for about a week, my karate teacher pulled me aside and said, "It's only pain. You worry too much about it." That brought me up short and made me think. My pain was real, yes, but I was too focused on it. I was letting it control my mood, using overt complaining about the pain to cover up my anger at myself for making an awkward move and my frustration at being slowed down, and then inflicting my bad mood on others with my whining. In a sense, I had abdicated control to the pain and made it worse than necessary.

Don't get me wrong. No one should have to put up with severe physical pain from disease and injury. In fact, we need to keep doing more, not less, in medicine to develop better pain management techniques and therapies. And my teacher's point shares a perception important in current pain management research: the emotional links to pain and how we understand those links may make all the difference between whether that pain is tolerable and manageable (and maybe even teaches us something) or whether it becomes a major distraction from what is really important in our lives.

In almost any circumstance, how we feel about what's happening— the emotions attached to or caused by those events—can either distract us and stop us cold or serve as a powerful and maturing force to help us move forward. In this chapter, we are going to look first at how the interconnectedness of the emotions and the physical body works to promote health or disease. Then we'll look at how some specific emotions and connections can either block us or support us in achieving high performance health. Those components that may distract us I call the "challenges," and those that can move us forward the "opportunities." In practice, emotions can sometimes be both challenges and opportunities, but it's useful to separate them for the purpose of discussion.

THE BIOLOGICAL POWER OF THE MIND— THE INTERFACE OF EMOTION AND HEALTH

In the previous chapter's discussion of how you can draw on the power of mind-body-spirit connections to create high performance thinking, I touched on the interface between our mental processes and our biological bodies. This field of study has often been called *psychobiology*, the biology of behavior. Thousands of scientific studies into dozens of aspects of this connection provide continually growing evidence of how what's in your head (brain) or in your heart (emotions) affects what happens in your body—and how what happens in your body affects what happens in your head and heart. We are discovering hundreds of links. Here are just a handful of examples that are relevant to the quest for high performance health.

- In one study conducted by Rippe Lifestyle Institute, walkers who adopted a mental strategy such as thinking pleasant thoughts while they were walking achieved significant reductions in anxiety and tension, as well as improvement in mood, compared to individuals who simply walked and did not have a mental strategy or who served as the control group.
- Numerous studies have shown that individuals who are under constant stress, who feel that they are not in control of their environment (air traffic controllers are a classic example), are at a much-increased risk of developing high blood pressure.[1]
- Numerous studies have shown that individuals who experience high levels of anger and frustration in their lives increase their risk of coronary artery disease, the leading killer of both men and women in the United States.[2]
- On the positive side, intriguing studies have shown that people who experience the love and support of others achieved better medical outcomes. For example, a study published by Dr. David Spiegel of the Stanford Medical School in the *Lancet* in 1989 compared two groups of women with metastatic breast cancer. These women were randomly divided into two groups, both of which received the same conventional medical therapies, such as surgery, radiation, medications, and chemotherapy, when indicated. In addition, one of the two groups met together ninety minutes each week for one year, during which time they were encouraged to talk about their illness in a supportive environment and express their feelings. These groups were led by a psychiatrist

and a social worker. The astounding result from this study was that the women in the group with the opportunity to talk about their feelings doubled their survival time![3]

While these are just a few examples, I can tell you that scientific literature concerning mind-body connections is enormous and growing every day. Failure to recognize the profound links between mind and body can prevent you from experiencing their beneficial power. If you acknowledge these connections, however, you can work to modify or heal those emotional responses or emotion-triggered behaviors that are blocking you and to draw on those that can strengthen you.

THE CHALLENGES

STRESS. We live in a stressful world. Any idea of eliminating stress from our lives is a fantasy. Eliminating stress may not even be desirable. A certain amount of stress helps us focus on achieving our goals. Stress becomes destructive or negative when it overwhelms our psychological and physiological capacity to constructively deal with it, neutralize it, or even benefit from it.

What exactly is stress? It's not an emotion. Broadly speaking, stress is any force that requires a response or change. For human beings, that response or change may be emotional or physiological or both. Where stress gets complicated, however, is that these emotional and physiological responses in turn may become stressors. For example, experiencing anxiety or fear or anger triggers the brain to release certain chemicals that signal the heart to beat faster and raise the blood pressure to prepare the body to fight the threat that triggered the emotion. Repeating this process frequently or continuously, as happens in our

> Failure to recognize the profound links between mind and body can prevent you from experiencing their beneficial power.

highly stressful modern environment, can overload the body's protective systems. The reverse is also true; what happens in the body's physiological systems can "stress" its emotional systems. For example, individuals who have experienced a heart attack frequently suffer from depression.

All the ways human biology and psychology interact are still far from clear, but the existence of such connections is not in doubt. Another consensus about stress that has emerged from extensive research is that the way in which we handle the many inevitable stressors in our lives in large measure determines whether the impact on our health and well-being will be neutral, negative, or maybe even positive. For example, my broken toe literally gave me greater pain while I was upset, frustrated, and unhappy about the situation than after I listened to my teacher and began to put my energies toward something other than complaining about myself.

> Stress becomes destructive or negative when it overwhelms our psychological and physiological capacity to constructively deal with it, neutralize it, or even benefit from it.

So how big a problem is stress? It's enormous. Based on epidemiological studies, an estimated half or more of all visits to physicians in the U.S. have a stress-related component; either stress contributes to the presenting illness or condition, or it is the primary complaint. A National Institutes of Health study showed that more than 30 percent of adults in the U.S. experience enough stress in their daily lives to hinder their performance either at home or at work.[4]

What about the links between stress and disease? Studies have shown that stress plays a role in conditions ranging all the way from cancer to the common cold. Stress is a significant contributor to high blood pressure and cardiac arrhythmias. Stress may play a role in the inflammatory response that contributes to the development of coronary artery disease. Stress can even contribute to dangerous arrhythmias that can lead to sudden cardiac death.

Here I want to make a crucial distinction between "stress" and "negative stress." Stress is something that all of us experience in our lives. It's only when we experience too much of it (without adequate coping strategies), attach a negative emotional overlay to it, or allow it to trigger potentially toxic emotions such as hostility, anger, hate, anxiety, fear, or shame that it becomes "negative stress."

Because stress plays such a central role in many issues of healing your emotions to revitalize your health, I'd like you to take a brief personal survey before you read the rest of this chapter. Your answers may alert you to some personal issues to keep in mind as you read and think through the rest of the chapter. This inventory has been adapted from the one we use at Rippe Health Assessment.

PERSONAL STRESS INVENTORY

How much job-related stress do you usually have?

Very little   Moderate amount   Quite a bit   Extreme amount

How much negative job-related stress do you usually experience?

Very little   Moderate amount   Quite a bit   Extreme amount

How do you feel you cope with your job-related stress?

Poorly   Fairly well   Moderately well   Very well

How much stress do you experience in your personal life?

Very little   Moderate amount   Quite a bit   Extreme amount

How much negative stress do you experience in your personal life?

Very little   Moderate amount   Quite a bit   Extreme amount

How well do you feel you cope with your personal stress?

Poorly   Fairly well   Moderately well   Very well

Do you have any symptoms that relate to your stress?

Yes   No

If yes, please list them:

_____

_____

_____

What does the inventory indicate about where you experience stress in your life and what kind of stress? Use the inventory as a springboard to think about areas where you may wish to work to reduce stress and areas where you cope well with stress. Record your thoughts in your journal.

The responses of the men and women who have undergone our Executive Health Evaluation may also interest you. More than 60 percent of our high-level executives experience quite a bit or extreme amounts of stress, but fewer than 50 percent report that stress as negative. Perhaps most important, when we ask individuals how well they cope with the stress at work, more than 70 percent respond that they cope either moderately well or very well. When we turn our attention to stress in these executives' personal lives, fewer than 20 percent experience quite a bit or extreme amounts of stress, and fewer than 15 percent experience that level of negative personal stress. An overwhelming 80 percent of individuals feel they cope moderately well or very well with stress in their personal lives.

Now, I know that this is an unusual population. High-level executives typically pride themselves in their ability to cope with stress. However, it is interesting to note that even these high achievers are experiencing high levels of stress. What seems to set them apart is not only their coping skills but also their ability to channel stress in such a way that it does not become negative in their personal lives.

Though stress is omnipresent, the good news is that we know a lot about how to manage it. One of the most effective ways is regular physical activity. For example, in a recent survey of individuals who exercised on a regular basis, more than 75 percent of respondents indicated that stress reduction was the major benefit of that exercise. As a cardiologist, I am very aware of the cardiovascular benefits that come from my regular exercise. Yet, as I told you earlier, the major reason I exercise daily is that I know it will give me more energy and reduce my stress. This is a secret that many high performance individuals have discovered. A few years ago when I surveyed many Fortune 500 CEOs, more than 60 percent of them indicated that they exercised at least three times a week, and the major reason they gave for doing this was stress reduction and enhancement of their performance. You can make this "secret" work for you.

> **Though stress is omnipresent, the good news is that we know a lot about how to manage it.**

There are many other techniques for relieving stress. Some of the best books for individuals on this subject have been written by Dr. Jon Kabat-Zinn, who ran the Mind-Body Stress Reduction program at the University of Massachusetts Medical School. His books on the role of meditation and stress reduction are excellent. I particularly recommend *Wherever You Go, There You Are: Mindfulness Meditation in Everyday Life* and *Full Catastrophe Living: Using the Wisdom of Your Body and Mind to Face Stress, Pain, and Illness.*[5]

As I have surveyed the literature on stress reduction, I believe it can be summarized in three concepts, which I have turned into a little rhyme to help me remember them:

- Seize the day.
- Get out of your own way.
- Make a personal play.

Seize the day. Remember to live in the present. Don't make the mistake of regretting the past or fearing the future—those behaviors just pile on stress. A fundamental tenet of stress reduction is to live in the present, or as I prefer to say, "seize the day."

Get out of your own way. Try not to add a negative emotional overlay to your stress. When I asked one CEO how he counseled his staff members to deal with their stress, he said, "I tell them not to worry that it is snowing outside; there is nothing you can do about the snow. You need to focus on those things you can handle and make a difference in, rather than focusing a lot of attention and worry on factors you can't control." He's certainly captured the core idea. The famous Serenity Prayer also helps many people: "God, grant me the serenity to accept the things I cannot change, the courage to change the things I can, and the wisdom to know the difference."

Make a personal play. Have a plan; don't leave stress free-floating. For many people, a "personal play"—a strategy taken from your personal playbook—can be as simple as being sure to walk every day. For others, it's meditating or spending time away from stressful circumstances. Each person will find specific techniques and strategies that help him or her manage and release stress.

ANGER. We live in a society that is not only stressed-out but also extremely angry. Although any day's news reports feature outbursts of violent anger erupting in shootings and killings, the anger endangering most of us is the anger that arises in response to day-to-day irritations, slights, and vexations. This type of anger is often veiled in behaviors we don't think of as anger, such as blaming or cynicism or even impatience. In *Anger Kills*, Dr. Redford Williams, a leading research scientist examining the health consequences of anger and hostility, compares such anger to "taking a small dose of some slow-acting poison—arsenic, for example—every day of your life."[6]

Failure to control the constant undercurrent of anger is hazardous to your health. How widespread are the anger hazards? An estimated 20 percent of Americans have anger levels high enough to present clear risk factors for disease; another 40 to 50 percent have enough anger to make their lives less satisfying and productive and potentially to harm their health.[7] The aspect of anger that appears to cause the greatest health risk is hostility. Anger also harms our relationships with others and tends to isolate us, circumstances that endanger our well-being. I might note that in my experience, resentment and hate also have ties to anger.

Failure to control the constant undercurrent of anger is hazardous to your health.

As with stress, however, there are many techniques to help you release and manage anger. Some of the stress-release techniques mentioned above also help with anger management. I have found that two simple techniques can help me avoid or defuse anger.

Ask of any anger-provoking situation, "Can I change it—is it in my control?" If the answer is no, then the only thing you can control is yourself. Release the irritation. For example, reckless and aggressive driving on the highway is a huge annoyance for many of us. But can we do anything to change the other drivers? Will getting steamed and frustrated change their behavior or simply cloud our better judgment? Practicing letting go of irritation and anger in such insignificant matters will help you defuse the impulse to anger in more important matters.

"No! Stop! Go away"—give yourself a personal time-out. Our oldest daughter at about three years old, while throwing a major tantrum, introduced what has become a very effective communication and anger management tool for our family. As only toddlers can, she was "pitching a fit." Determined to defuse the situation, I asked her to give me a hug. "No!" she responded. "How about a kiss?" I gently countered. "Stop!" she yelled, turning away. I finally went for one of our favorite routines "Then give me a high five." She whirled around, looked me square in the eyes, and said, "Go AWAY!" It was clear that she was

determined to have her own process for stopping the tantrum rather than yield to my intervention. And she did work her way out of it.

As we laughed, then reflected on this encounter, Stephanie and I realized that our daughter had given us a valuable lesson about communicating and managing our angry emotions. Though acting out, our daughter was essentially giving herself a time-out. In the years since, our family has used this technique to avoid potentially explosive arguments and to enhance communication. Of course, I'm not recommending that as an adult you use a toddler's literal words— "No! Stop! Go away" but that you recognize the value of clearly communicating your need to cool down and your intention of taking a personal time-out until you can bring calm thoughts and actions to a discussion of the issue.

An excellent resource for further exploring anger management is *Anger Kills* by Dr. Redford Williams and his wife, Virginia Williams, PhD. In addition to describing the adverse consequences of uncontrolled anger and hostility, the Drs. Williams provide a very compelling road map for dealing with anger. As you pursue high performance health, I particularly recommend their strategies that involve trusting others, trying to be empathetic, and practicing forgiveness.

ANXIETY AND DEPRESSION. Stress also plays a role in two common problems in our society: anxiety and depression. Anxiety is typically characterized by exaggerated worry and tension often about everyday matters. Depression has many manifestations but generally can involve feelings of worthlessness, meaninglessness, hopelessness, emptiness, or anxiety. In addition to the millions who have anxiety disorders or clinical depression, many people suffer from some of the emotions associated with anxiety or depression. When a patient comes to me with a complaint of fatigue, for example, I check for anxiety and depression as potential underlying causes of the fatigue. Of course, I always check for potential underlying medical conditions such as a low blood count or poor physical conditioning, but in many instances, anxiety or depression turns out to be the cause for fatigue.

I mention the potential challenges of anxiety and depression in this chapter because I want you to be aware of them. And I want to assure you that if you are experiencing any of the feelings or outlooks associated with anxiety or depression, you can do something about them.

> Studies show that individuals who set realistic goals and then take specific actions to accomplish those goals . . . often get the added psychological benefit of reduced anxiety and depression.

Our research team at Rippe Lifestyle Institute, for example, has published numerous studies on the effects of regular physical activity and weight loss on anxiety and depression. These studies show that individuals who set realistic goals and then take specific actions to accomplish those goals, whether they be weight loss, better nutrition, or increased physical activity, often get the added psychological benefit of reduced anxiety and depression.

If you are experiencing ongoing symptoms associated with anxiety or depression, you should consult your physician and ask for a thorough evaluation. I would also encourage you to work with your physician to create a balanced therapeutic plan for you. There is certainly a role for both psychotherapy and medication to relieve anxiety and depression, but too often, I am convinced, we opt first for medications for these conditions and overlook the benefits of lifestyle measures, such as planning and carrying out regular physical activity. Here's one area where you can help take back control of your health with support from your physician.

PAIN AND GRIEF. Hurt and grief carry burdens of pain that strike deep inside. To believe that you can avoid pain in your life is not realistic. Part of deriving the joy and comfort of relationships with others is accepting the reality that these relationships will also bring distress and great sadness. Inevitably, hurts will occur as life goes along, and there will be losses. Some losses may arise from behaviors and hurts within relationships. The last inevitable loss comes in death.

Loss is traumatic. Loss not only wounds our spirits but also stresses our bodies. Sometimes hurt and loss may be mixed up with anger or anxiety. The pain inside "where the meanings are" can seem over-whelming. Emily Dickinson captured this sensation in just a few lines:

Pain—has an Element of Blank—
It cannot recollect
When it begun—or if there were
A time when it was not.

As the "Blank" disappears, however, other emotions begin to play a role. Anger may become mixed with fear or guilt. Isolation may seem to loom. In periods of hurt or despair, doing anything for yourself, such as working for high performance health, may seem worthless.

This may be the time to remind yourself that pain is one of the prices we pay for being full and whole human beings. How can we really know safety and security when we have them unless we know loss? As Bruce Springsteen sings, "The feeling of safety you prize / Well, it comes with a hard hard price."[8]

I am also reminded of how one may turn pain to positive purpose by one of our family's favorite scenes in *The Lion King*. Happy in his carefree, self-imposed exile, the young lion Simba encounters his old playmate Nala, who tells him about the desolation of the Pridelands and urges him to return home to his rightful duties as leader of the pride. The idea scares Simba; he still feels terrible guilt at causing the death of his father and fears responsibility. At this point, the wise elder Rafiki whacks the unsuspecting Simba on the head with his staff. Simba yelps at the pain, protesting. Rafiki replies, "You can do two things with your pain—you can run from it or you can learn from it."

If we would achieve our best health and live fully, then we must learn from our pain. It's at times of hurt and pain that you need high performance thinking and activity most. Give yourself some space, permission to grieve and to cry. There is nothing weak about grieving for genuine loss. Then reach out to your partnerships for support (you identified those strengths in Chapter 4). I also recommend that, even if you are "just going through the motions," you take your daily walk or do another physical activity. Research shows that physical activity can help our spirits heal.

> If we would achieve our best health and live fully, then we must learn from our pain.

DENIAL. Denial is one of the most dangerous emotional responses to life. Denial is a behavior that may arise from a complex of emotional factors including anxiety, fear, guilt, depression, and other motivators. It can contribute in very significant ways to harming our health because often we are in denial about behaviors that pose known health risks. Another trap about denial—it's often easy to recognize in others but much harder to see in our own behavior.

I observed one of the most startling examples when I was in medical school, when I had the privilege of scrubbing in with top thoracic surgeons during my surgical rotation. Now, the 1970s was a different era in medicine, but it was well-known even then that cigarette smoking represented a significant risk factor for lung cancer. Nonetheless, one of the senior thoracic surgeons, after spending hours in the operating room removing aggressive lung tumors in smokers, would step outside after each case and smoke a cigarette. Now, I know cigarette smoking is extremely addictive, but clearly this senior surgeon was also in denial of his own mortality and the incredible risk that he was taking by continuing to smoke a pack a day. This, despite removing lung tumors in patients on a daily basis! As my medical experience grew, I came to know that such denial is a human failing.

Denial in cardiac patients can be deadly. The American Heart Association spends an enormous amount of time and energy each year trying to convince people that when they have symptoms suggestive of a heart attack or impending stroke, they need to call 911 immediately and get to an emergency room so that therapy can be initiated. Yet despite this, many people linger in unsafe environments, such as their home, denying that they are having symptoms of a heart attack or a stroke. In one famous case reported in the *New England Journal of Medicine*, a man actually ran up and down the stairs at a hotel and did push-ups when he was having chest pain to determine whether or not he was having a heart attack! The good news is, he managed to survive this folly and lived to tell the tale.

> By making a conscientious effort to make small changes in your daily life, you can get out of this pattern of denial and experience the good health that we all want and deserve.

Subtler forms of denial can certainly harm your health. As I've pointed out before, almost all adults know physical inactivity or being overweight or obese increases their risk of chronic disease. But a majority of us continue to live in denial, easing our minds by indulging in the Tomorrow Promise. You know:

"I'll start walking tomorrow, after the company leaves."

"I'll start a weight-loss program after the stress of completing this project is over or after the holidays when the food's not so tempting."

"I'll start planning for high performance health tomorrow."

Unfortunately, the Tomorrow Promise never works, as Alice in Wonderland realized when she said, "It's always jam yesterday or jam tomorrow, never jam today." The "jam," not a sugary treat but a healthy pleasure, that I want for you *today* is to stop fooling yourself and make a small step toward change. By making a conscientious effort to make small changes in your daily life, you can get out of this pattern of denial and experience the good health that we all want and deserve.

Sometimes comfortable in denial, we convince ourselves that we have achieved all we need. In one of his last poems, my friend Rad Smith captured this feeling that we may have built "the perfect house," but he goes on to challenge us to make more of our opportunities:

> Build the perfect house, then burn it down
> every vaulted ceiling, the vitrine
> of skeleton clocks, the stained
> glass window. You can do better.[9]

THE OPPORTUNITIES

As I have matured as a physician and person and had the opportunity to share wonderful and, yes, at times heartbreaking experiences with my patients, I have come to understand that emotions can not only hinder our health and life but can also be a source of great power and blessing. In this section, we look at some of those opportunities.

LOVE. The capacity to love and be loved is a cornerstone value for high performance health and high performance living. Love is so vast, multifaceted, and mysterious that it defies definition. But I can share a few perceptions of what about love is so important to achieving high performance health and living fully.

When we love, we give of the best of ourselves. When we are loved unconditionally as God loves us, we are freed to stretch and keep growing in love for ourselves and for others and growing in so many other ways. When we love, we open ourselves up to great joy and happiness as well as to vulnerability, pain, and grief—we give ourselves the possibility of being fully realized human beings. Love is, as Thornton Wilder observed, "the bridge between the land of the living and the land of the dead"—in particular, love is our bridge from the deadly stagnation of indifference to caring about being fully alive. At one level, pursuing high performance health is an exploration of what it means to love yourself and do the best for yourself so that you can better love and support those you hold dearest.

Many of the opportunities I will discuss in the next pages are made possible in some way by love. If you'd like to explore the role of love in health and healing and spiritual growth beyond the few ideas I can share here, I recommend three insightful books. An early work in this field, Dr. Bernie Siegel's *Love, Medicine and Miracles,* makes the case for the healing power of love. In *The Road Less Traveled,* Dr. M. Scott Peck, who is a

> Emotions can not only hinder our health and life but can also be a source of great power and blessing.

psychiatrist and man of faith, explores the role of love in lifelong spiritual growth. Dr. Dean Ornish in *Love and Survival* documents multiple scientific studies showing health benefits from love.

CONNECTEDNESS AND COMMUNITY. One of the best ways to give and experience love, acceptance, and support is by nurturing our connectedness and sense of community with others. Numerous studies have shown that individuals who feel connected with other human beings and who are members of a community improve both their health and likelihood of survival compared to individuals who feel socially isolated. For example, in one study conducted by Dr. Redford Williams at Duke University, fourteen hundred men and women who were diagnosed by coronary catheterization with at least one significant narrowing in a coronary artery were followed for five years. At the end of that time, individuals who were not married or did not have at least one close confidant were three times as likely to have died as those who were married or had a confidant or both. Numerous other studies have shown similar findings.[10]

You might assume that in our increasingly "wired" world, people would be more likely to establish connections with other people. Sadly, the opposite has occurred. In 1985, the average American had three people in whom they could confide matters important to them. By 2004, the average number of close confidants had dropped to two, and one in four people had no close confidants. Robert Putnam documents this disturbing trend toward social isolation in his book *Bowling Alone*. A key component of achieving high performance health, however, is to follow the words from an old AT&T ad campaign, "Reach out and touch someone." Spending the time and effort to establish close connections with others not only increases pleasure and meaning in life but actually benefits your health.

> Spending the time and effort to establish close connections with others not only increases pleasure and meaning in life but actually benefits your health.

SPIRITUALITY. One of the ways that we connect to others is through our spirits. Our spirits are vital to fulfilling lives. Yet many of us neglect the importance of taking care of our spiritual health. I believe caring for our spirits is fundamental to caring for our health. I agree with Thomas Moore when he writes:

> The great malady of the twentieth century implicated in all of our troubles and affecting us individually and socially is loss of soul. When soul is neglected, it doesn't just go away; it appears symptomatically in obsessions, addiction, violence and loss of meaning. Our temptation is to try to isolate these symptoms or try to eradicate them one by one; but the root problem is that we have lost our wisdom about the soul, even our interest in it.[11]

As a remedy to this diagnosis, I urge the careful cultivation and nurturing of the spirit, which will yield multiple and important health benefits that spill over into virtually every aspect of your life. Both Scott

Peck's *The Road Less Traveled* and Thomas Moore's *Care of the Soul* will challenge and inspire your thinking.

PURPOSE. At the beginning of this book, I described a values-driven approach linking health to fitness, performance, appearance, joy, and meaning. Meaning and purpose are inextricably linked. The quest for purpose is dynamic because life is a journey and not a destination. You may have discovered your overall purpose for your journey on the planet, but finding the itinerary is ongoing.

When I was in college, I was introduced to the power of purpose through many great orators, including the late Martin Luther King Jr. While everyone remembers Dr. King's famous "I have a dream" speech, in which he laid out his vision for the future of racial harmony in America, I was equally struck by a speech he gave in June 1963, when he rallied his volunteers who were discouraged by the difficulty of creating change through nonviolence. Dr. King was talking about how the volunteers should respond to those who attacked them. He stated of nonviolence that "if he [the opponent] puts you in jail, you go in that jail and transform it from a dungeon of shame to a haven of freedom and human dignity. And even if he tries to kill you, you'll develop the inner conviction that there are some things so dear, some things so precious, some things so eternally true, that they are worth dying for. And I submit to you that if a man has not discovered something that he will die for, he isn't fit to live."[12] It would be hard to find a clearer statement about why it's important to discover purpose.

> Caring for our spirit is fundamental to caring for our health.

HOPE. One of my favorite passages of Scripture is 1 Corinthians 13, where the apostle Paul counseled the Corinthians that "faith, hope and love abide, these three; but the greatest of these is love" (Vo 13 NRSV). I have already spoken about faith (as trust) and love; the third quality of *hope* is also one of the touchstones of emotional health. Hope has much in common with optimism and vision.

Hope, along with passion, energized Marla's quest for health and healing. I first saw Marla when she and her husband arrived for health evaluations more than five years ago. Although Marla had not smoked for fifteen years and felt fine, she previously had smoked more than a pack a day. Our clinic was among the first to offer high-speed CT scanning for early diagnosis of certain diseases. With Marla's history of smoking, therefore, we ordered a preventive lung scan, which, unfortunately, detected a localized lung cancer. Fortunately, the screening led to early detection. Marla engaged totally in her treatment plan, partnering with her health-care team. Along with surgery to remove the tumor and follow-up radiation therapy, Marla immersed herself in scientific literature related to cancer and nutrition, and she added an exercise program as recommended. Anchored in hope and supported by her family, Marla looked and worked forward. She focused on living. After more than five years, she has had no recurrence of the lung cancer and has *enjoyed* life.

Marla's deep hope and belief for the future were her ally in her fight against cancer. Hope can be your ally as you work toward achieving your best health now.

FORGIVENESS. It is very difficult to truly forgive people who may have insulted or wronged us in some way. Yet practicing true forgiveness is a powerful way to revitalize your health and well-being. Letting go of injury and insult, relaxing your grip on internal wounds, is like loosing the shackles that have bound you to those injuries. It is also important to seek forgiveness and let go of guilt when you feel you may have hurt someone else. It's no overstatement to say forgiveness is critically important to your health and essential to a fully realized life.

In his book *The Return of the Prodigal Son*, Henri Nouwen shares his deep reflections on the biblical parable of the prodigal son as seen through the lens of his contemplation of Rembrandt's painting of the son's return. In the parable, the younger son of a well-to-do man, tired of working in the family business, comes to his father and requests his share of his future inheritance right then. The father grants this wish. Happily flush with money, the son leaves for a foreign country, where he leads a life of leisure and debauchery. He quickly burns through all of his inheritance and ends up in desperate straits. Finally, he realizes the error of his ways and thinks of all he has turned his back on at home, where even the lowliest servant is well cared for. Filled with remorse, the prodigal returns to his father, begging for forgiveness and a place in his home as a servant. His father freely grants this forgiveness and even throws a celebratory feast, much to the dismay and resentment of the older, dutiful son, who feels his father should punish the younger son for his transgressions.[13]

> Forgiveness is critically important to your health and essential to a fully realized life.

Nouwen beautifully describes how all of us are called upon to forgive each other, much in the way God has forgiven us. A key part of this in Nouwen's explanation is that first we must learn to forgive ourselves and each other and truly believe we are worthy of being "found" and forgiven by God. Most of us struggle mightily with learning how to forgive freely and fully without conditions, but the health benefits of practicing forgiveness are enormous.

Another very useful book on this subject is my friend Dick Tibbits's *Forgive to Live*, in which he makes the case that a muscular forgiveness is a cornerstone of good health, both physical and spiritual.

THE IMPORTANCE OF HEALING

Healing and health are related but different. *Healing* is a verb and implies action, whereas *health* is a noun and refers to a state of being. Healing is an active process we all can participate in, whether or not we are faced with specific physical health challenges. The good news is that our bodies possess an enormous and renewable capability to heal. Even if you are faced with health challenges, if you apply the principles we discuss in this book, you will find new ways to allow your body to work with you to truly achieve not only health but healing.

I went into medicine because I viewed it as a healing art. I saw it as a way of taking action to improve people's lives. As medicine has evolved into the complicated alphabet soup of PPOs, HMOs, EOBs, and the like, there is a constant danger of drifting farther and farther away from the healing art of medicine. Guarding against this drift is one reason I have urged you to establish a partnership with your physician. Healing is a process in which your actions and thoughts are probably more important than anything your doctor can do—although, in a true partnership, you get the best of both. Healing, in my view, also involves the laying on of hands. I truly believe in the healing power of touch. After all, Christ often healed people by first placing His hands on them. Drawing on all your resources for healing, therefore, means tapping into the power of mind-body-spirit connections in partnership with the best resources of modern medicine.

> No matter what your health challenges are, you can play an important role in your own healing process.

No matter what your health challenges are, you can play an important role in your own healing process. In fact, many of my patients with very significant chronic illnesses derive enormous benefits from the types of emotional opportunities we have discussed in this chapter.

HEALING AND AGING About a decade ago, I wrote a book called *Fit over Forty*, discussing what I had discovered about fitness and health as I began to work my way through my forties. Now that I am in my fifties, I look back at this book and my perceptions then. I was determined that the "autumn" of my own life would, in John Berryman's words, "come as a prize." That is still my goal. I still embrace the importance of sound nutrition, healthy weight management, and regular exercise. But some of my specific fitness targets have changed: I swim more and run less, and when I run, the young exercise physiologists and my research director, Dr. Ted Angelopoulos, have to slow their running pace so we can run together. I would like to say I have solved most of the issues and problems I identified ten years ago, but the journey continues, and I discover that this continuing exploration is also a prize.

In some ways my view of healing has changed and matured. Part of this is the simple fact of growing older. I am sure part of this also relates to becoming the father of four beautiful and active children. Nonetheless, my view of emotional well-being and the power of my mind to help heal my body have deepened considerably over the past decade. My life is richer, and my experience is deeper than ever before, but I find I agree with T. S. Eliot's perception: "As we grow older / The world seems stranger, the pattern more complicated / Of dead and living."[14]

I certainly see the pattern as even more complicated than I did just ten years ago. However, one of the great blessings of aging is that we begin to shed some of the ambiguities of youth and focus at a deeper level on some of the key challenges of health and living. I am trying to drink deeply from life. Many times I do; sometimes I don't. I accept that life is often two steps forward and one step back. Nonetheless, I am determined that the pursuit of what Eliot calls a "deeper union, a further communion" will continue to be the highest priority of my life. And that priority undergirds my determination to continue to promote my own health as a tool for high performance living. I urge you to think about your health in the same way, regardless of what age you are.

GENERATIONS

When I was an undergraduate in college, I had the pleasure of studying with the great psychologist Erik Erikson. Professor Erikson had developed a framework describing the stages of normal human development all of us experience in our lives. The last stage of development, which he candidly discussed in his lectures, he called "generativity versus despair." He described this as the time toward the end of each person's life when he or she either tries to pass on important lessons to the next generation or lapse into despair. I am determined that the latter portions of my own life be filled with generativity. Each of us owes this gift to the next generation. And if we engage in lovingly passing on our knowledge, enthusiasm, and wisdom to the next generation, remarkably, the effort and connection will not only benefit our lives with added meaning and health but will also be enormously beneficial for the health and well-being of our children and grandchildren.

> Many of the issues we have discussed about healing your own emotions to revitalize your health also can be passed on to your children.

Two important studies have shown the value of loving relationships between parents and children for the health of the children. (I would hypothesize the same kinds of benefits for connections between grandparent and grandchildren.)

In one study from the Johns Hopkins Medical School, more than one thousand male medical students completed a test that assessed the students' perception of their relationship with their parents. The individuals surveyed were then followed for up to fifty years later. Clear distinctions among groups emerged. Those men who had reported caring relationships and perceived themselves to be loved by their parents were significantly less likely to develop chronic diseases such as cancer than were their classmates who had more negative perceptions of their relationships with their parents.[15]

In a similar study performed among Harvard medical students in the 1950s, students who felt that they were loved by their parents were significantly less likely in subsequent follow-up over the next forty years to develop various chronic illnesses.[16]

Thus, many of the issues we have discussed about healing your own emotions to revitalize your health also can be passed on to your children.

A FURTHER WORD ABOUT PARTNERING WITH YOUR PHYSICIAN

When it comes to healing, many of the issues we have discussed in this chapter are sadly lacking in health care in the U.S. today. Your physician may even resist some of the ideas expressed in this book about the power of love, spirituality, connectedness, and purpose when it comes to improving health. I urge you to be patient with your doctor. There is so much to learn in medical school that oftentimes people leave without a fundamental understanding of the vast literature supporting the powerful relationships between mind and body and the important role of emotions in health and healing.

As we travel down the path toward high performance health, each of us will struggle to turn our emotions into a powerful force for good health in our lives; yet the journey is incredibly meaningful.

MAKING IT PERSONAL

To reflect on this chapter, consider the following questions and record your reflections and goals in your journal.

Please list any emotional "challenges" you have and outline ways you are going to work to overcome them.

List emotional opportunities that exist in your life to improve your health and list how you are going to take advantage of them.

_____

_____

_____

_____

_____

List some ways you can participate in your own healing process and specific actions you will take to enhance these.

_____

_____

_____

_____

_____

7 | STOP TO REST AND HEAL WHEN YOUR BODY AND SPIRIT NEED IT

Sleep that knits up the ravell'd sleeve of care,
The death of each day's life, sore labour's bath,
Balm of hurt minds, great nature's second course,
Chief nourisher in life's feast.

—WILLIAM SHAKESPEARE, *MACBETH*

I loafe and invite my soul,
I lean and loafe at my ease observing a spear
  of summer grass.

—WALT WHITMAN, *SONG OF MYSELF*

Rest and healing are two critically important parts of achieving your best possible health. Rest provides time for your body to heal from the daily damage inflicted by the stresses of living. Rest rejuvenates your energy and spirit. You can't achieve true healing without allowing the body to work with you: rest provides that opportunity. Rest and healing literally keep us alive.

Yet both rest and healing are undervalued in our society and in our health-care system. For example, multitasking is widely considered an important skill for success. How often have you been talking on the phone with one person while e-mailing another or participating in a business meeting while text-messaging a colleague? How about negotiating highway traffic while talking on your cell phone? We brag about how much activity we can cram into a single day, and some businesses even list "multitasking" among the skills required in a job candidate. Yet research suggests that by multitasking, we actually accomplish less work, and certainly less quality work, than we would if we focused on tasks sequentially and used our technology to help us do that. So multitasking ramps up our stress while lowering our achievement. That's not a high performance value. As Jared Sandberg observed recently in a *Wall Street Journal* column, "What now passes for multitasking was once called not paying attention."[1] We pay physically and spiritually for the pressure of dividing ourselves in too many directions.

> We pay physically and spiritually for the pressure of dividing ourselves in too many directions.

The chances are good, too, that neither your physician nor other health-care professionals will offer you a course correction. One reason most physicians have difficulty discussing the value of rest with their patients lies in the intensive training schedules of most internships and residencies. I can remember the two-year period when I was on call every third night in addition to working all day. I was so busy taking care of patients that I rarely got to sleep. Although the hospital provided "sleep rooms" for the residents on call, my colleagues and I seldom got the chance to stretch out. In fact, we laughed at the black humor of an essay entitled "On Sleep" posted in one sleep room because we did so little of it. Such intensive training experience certainly provides firsthand knowledge of many more medical conditions than most physicians would otherwise encounter, but the knowledge comes at a cost.

This attitude of undervaluing rest also tends to be institutionalized in medical instruction. Let me give you an example. One major internal medicine textbook, which is used in virtually every medical school in the United States and is the go-to reference for practicing physicians, has twenty-two hundred pages of small-print entries on almost every known disease. Yet this huge textbook provides not one entry devoted to "rest." The closest the discussion comes to considering rest is one paragraph devoted to "relaxation." Even then, relaxation is discussed only as a risk factor for insomnia. And what about healing? After all, medicine is a healing art. Again, there is no entry for "healing" in this or any other major internal medicine textbook I have examined.

This lack of emphasis on rest and healing reflects a fundamental problem in American medicine: we don't recognize the importance of the restorative process for good health. All of us, including health-care professionals and individuals who want to take personal charge of their health, need to reframe how we think about the restorative processes that foster good health.

ACTIVE REST

The first thing you need to know about rest is that it's not a passive condition but an active time when your body is working to regenerate and rejuvenate itself. Too often people mistake resting for laziness or lack of discipline. Just the opposite is true. Walt Whitman captured the essence of rest, I think, when he wrote, "I loafe and invite my soul." Rest that invites you to explore new dimensions certainly isn't laziness. And making time to rest both your body and your soul in your busy daily life surely takes discipline.

Active rest will take different forms for different people. Your challenge will be first to find how your body really rests and then to provide time for rest. For example, my concentration starts to lag after forty-five minutes of work, so I make it a point to get up and do something different for ten minutes every hour, if at all possible. Of course, meetings and/or family obligations sometimes prevent this from happening, but when I'm working solo, I am more productive if I relax for ten minutes

Rest helps your body repair its structures at all levels.

every hour. I may play with one of my dogs, stroll around the garden, make myself a latte, or do a small task. I also exercise for forty-five minutes to an hour every day. This is a period of disciplined rest in my life. It may seem illogical that my exercise time is a "rest" time, but these sessions take me away from current work or problems and let me relax. As a result, some of my best thinking and problem solving occurs during these exercise sessions. Sometimes you must expend energy in order to gain energy.

Now, I am not saying that everyone needs to exercise every day or even use exercise as a time of rest and relaxation. In fact, many people prefer reading a book or listening to music or tending their garden. I know of one highly productive businessman who insists that the secret to his high energy in addition to a regular exercise program is his ability to take ten-minute "power naps" whenever the need strikes, often in midafternoon. The point is to figure out what works in your life and take disciplined periods of rest periodically throughout the day. Of course, nighttime rest, including sleep, is also critically important to the healing process.

Whatever your techniques, active rest has five components:

- Repair
- Sleep
- Retreat
- Relax
- Actively recover

REPAIR. When you've worked hard physically or mentally for hours, you know how refreshing it can be to kick back in your easy chair or slip onto the couch for a quick snooze. While we experience such restorative rest on the macro level, this restorative process is also active at the micro level of our bodies' cells. Both the body's normal metabolic processes and environmental threats such as UV radiation damage the DNA molecules that record the genetic information in our cells. Daily, every cell in our bodies experiences from one thousand to one million molecular "lesions," damage that needs repair. Left unrepaired, such damage can lead to numerous diseases, including cancers and various autoimmune disorders, and to the aging process itself.

Rest provides our cells time to repair DNA. Consequently, it's vital that we reduce the stresses caused by nonstop activity, exposure to toxic environments, and destructive habits, such as overeating and smoking in order to give our cells times to repair themselves. Each cell has an enormous capacity to repair itself if we remove enough stress to allow the natural processes to occur.

Rest helps your body repair its structures at all levels. For instance, when you strength train to build more muscle—a strategy that helps keep your metabolism high as you lose or maintain weight—the muscle grows by a process of minute tears during exercise and recovery and healing during rest. That's why physiologists recommend that we perform strength-training exercises every other day rather than every day.

SLEEP. Most of us would agree with Shakespeare's view of sleep as a "balm" that "knits up the raveled sleeve of care" or the "chief nourisher in life's feast." Numerous studies have shown that most adults need seven to eight hours of sleep for optimal functioning. But the average American gets fewer than seven hours of sleep on weeknights, many far fewer. Regularly sleeping fewer than five hours or more than nine hours a night is associated with poorer health profiles.

An estimated one-third of American adults (more than 70 million people) have difficulty sleeping, at least on occasion. Other industrialized nations report similar statistics. Insomnia is also common, particularly in older people. In fact, an estimated 15 to 20 percent of people age fifty-five and older report sleep problems great enough to harm their quality of life.[2]

The problem of sleep deprivation is real. Unfortunately, our tendency to reach immediately for drug therapy to treat sleep problems is probably not the most effective answer. As a society, however, we love the "quick fix," and pharmaceutical companies have been happy to flood the market with newly developed sleep aids. In addition, hospital-trained physicians may gravitate first toward medical solutions because they learned about sleep in hospital settings, where many people have difficulty sleeping and sleep-promoting medications are often appropriate. Yet in everyday life, most individuals who are having trouble sleeping may actually get greater help from a variety of behavioral strategies.

I recommend that you try some of these proven behavioral strategies to enhance your sleeping patterns before you ask your physician for a prescription.

Adopt positive lifestyle activities that enhance sleep. For instance, get regular physical activity during the day, but avoid exercising right before bedtime. A nutritious, balanced diet is also helpful. Avoiding spicy foods and caffeinated beverages for dinner or within two or three hours of bedtime may reduce problems that prevent falling asleep. Also avoid alcohol late; it may make you drowsy, but it also inhibits aspects of sleep that let you sleep soundly through the night.

Keep to a sleep schedule. If you are having trouble sleeping, it helps to schedule the time you go to bed and the time you get up—and keep to your schedule. The point is to make sleep a habit. It may take some days to establish your routine, so even if you don't fall asleep quickly when you go to bed, continue to arise at your scheduled time.

Control sleep-preventing stimuli. Make sure you use your bedroom for sleep and not for activities incompatible with sleeping, such as eating, playing loud music, or in many cases, watching television. Think about adjusting such environmental factors as noise, temperature, and light to make your bedroom more conducive to rest and sleep.

Learn relaxation techniques. Learning how to relax can help you "fall into" sleep. You may find a relaxation program on tape or CD or deep-breathing techniques helpful. Here's a simple technique that works for many: as you lie in a comfortable position, visualize the progressive relaxation of your body, starting with your toes. As you focus on your feet, intentionally relax them, letting them sink more comfortably into the bed each time you breathe out. Move smoothly up to your lower and upper legs, your hips, your torso. Push intrusive thoughts gently away as you focus on breathing and relaxing. Gradually, you should drift into sleep.

> Sleep is active rest that charges up the body for optimal functioning.

Consider cognitive therapy. Some people may have fears or beliefs that interfere with their ability to sleep. Cognitive therapy can often help individuals learn to think differently about sleep and to replace the blocks with realistic expectations.

Sleep is active rest that charges up the body for optimal functioning. For example, getting enough sleep helps us focus better, think and react more quickly, and do better at creative problem solving. During sleep, we also experience a variety of hormonal changes that reset our "time clocks" and help determine how our bodies use energy. Individuals who get too little sleep have higher risks of high blood pressure, heart disease, diabetes, and overweight. For all these reasons, sleep is good for your body and soul. It's critical to achieving high performance health.

RETREAT. Disciplined periods away from the stresses of your current situation also promote proper rest. My friend Bill Morgan, who has published important studies in this area, calls planned periods away from the stressors of daily life "time-outs." Regular daily exercise can be a powerful restorative habit in part because it provides a disciplined time-out.

In addition to such daily time-outs, however, you need longer periods of retreat and escape. For example, a man I'll call Roger, who is the chairman of one of the largest companies in the United States, takes one day a month away from work. During that day off, he refuses to answer e-mail or phone calls or have any other communication with the numerous people who constantly demand his time. Roger asserts that these disciplined monthly retreats help him maintain the focus and fast pace required of a senior executive in a very large company.

As the senior executive of your own busy life, I suggest you plan regular one-day or longer retreats to help you regroup, reenergize, refocus, and relax. Earlier we saw the benefits of setting aside one day each week as a Sabbath rest for your body and spirit. In addition, I urge you to consider taking an extended vacation at least once a year.

However, let me give you a word of caution about vacations. Be sure to view your vacations not as times to pack in a lot of activities, but rather as opportunities for spiritual and physical rejuvenation. How many times have you heard people returning from vacations say,

> I suggest you plan regular one-day or longer retreats to help you regroup, refocus, reenergize, and relax.

"I need a vacation from my vacation!" Stephanie and I have often been guilty of this. But we have learned that our best retreats come when our family slips away to a secluded place in the mountains. We dip our feet in the river. We walk in the woods. We genuinely enjoy one another's company without any pressure to see other people or fulfill any social obligations. It took us a long time to recognize that what we love to do the most is be with one another, away from the demands of the world. I challenge you to find what types of retreats bring you restoration.

RELAX. Relaxation enables optimum performance. Although we associate maximum effort and extraordinary skills with the highest levels of athletic performance, relaxation may actually be the critical element that separates the champions from the merely great.

I learned this many years ago when I was on a speaking tour with Jackie Joyner-Kersee, whom *Sports Illustrated* named the all-time best female athlete. In the late eighties, Jackie had recently won her first gold medal in the Olympic heptathlon, seven events blending strength, speed, and endurance. Jackie's great strength was her jumping, but she had to work at the speed events such as the 200-meter and 800-meter runs. She said the final breakthrough for her in these speed events came when her coach convinced her of the importance of relaxing in order to run faster. Jackie Joyner-Kersee still holds the world record in heptathlon with the six best results in history. (She also accomplished this despite exertion-induced asthma.)

> We need to approach all rest as "active recovery" that assists our bodies in getting rid of toxic waste products, whether they be physical or emotional, and enables healing to take place.

Joe Montana has described the same phenomenon of relaxing to perform at your best. Joe was famous for his almost mystical calmness during periods of high stress. For example, during a television time-out in the last two minutes of a Super Bowl game, while Joe was leading his team for the potential winning score, he spotted actor John Candy on the sidelines and pointed him out to his teammates. They were amazed at his calmness. But Joe asserts that staying on an even keel, never getting too high or too low, is critical to performance.

I recently discovered for myself how important relaxation can be to performance in my "new" sport of swimming. Most fiftysomethings don't take up the butterfly stroke and expect to excel. but living with a family of swimmin' women, I was determined to do my best. I worked and worked up and down the pool lane, but I really struggled until I realized the secret to the butterfly stroke was to pull strongly while my arms were under the water and to relax and recover on the arc out of the water.

Once I learned to relax, my style and my speed increased—and those mutterings about "windmills in water" ceased.

Relaxing, like resting, is an active process. You must consciously think about letting go of mental and physical tension as you experience them. Practice keeping an even keel and working with your body and not against it. Staying relaxed enhances your performance whatever you are doing.

ACTIVELY RECOVER. Athletes have known for many years the importance not only of warming up prior to an exercise session but also of cooling down afterward. That's why, for instance, you see runners at track meets walking or jogging slowly after they have finished the race. Such "active recovery" after exercise allows the body to more efficiently rid itself of waste products generated during exercise.

In a broader sense, we need to approach all rest as "active recovery" that assists our bodies in getting rid of toxic waste products, whether they be physical or emotional, and enables healing to take place.

HEALING

Healing is at the core of high performance health. We need healing not just when we are sick or injured, but all the time. I've already discussed the millions of "hits" our DNA takes daily. Because our bodies and spirits are subject to continuous hits, healing also must be continuous.

As captain of your high performance health team, you play an important role in enhancing healing. This is true whether you are facing a specific health challenge or simply trying to move from good health to high performance health. Numerous studies have shown that when individuals participate fully in the healing process, no matter their health challenges, they can achieve superior outcomes.

Many of the therapies available through medicine are really designed to help the body repair itself. For example, in cardiac rehabilitation, we use exercise programs and nutritional changes to help strengthen the heart as part of the recovery process for an individual who has suffered a heart attack. But comprehensive cardiac rehabilitation also involves supporting the individual's spiritual and emotional healing.

When I think about this view of healing, I often think of Walt. At age forty-three, Walt had suffered a major heart attack and continued to have significant chest pain (angina) with even minimal exertion. He had been referred to me for consultation and a heart catheterization. Walt's wife, Sheila, and his two young children accompanied him into my office. Walt came right to the point. He was dejected that his own actions, such as smoking, in-activity, and weight gain, had probably contributed signifi-cantly to the early develop-

> When individuals participate fully in the healing process, no matter what health challenges they face, they can achieve superior outcomes.

ment of his coronary artery disease. He felt guilty and depressed and hopeless. I assured him there was no reason to give up hope. What had happened, had happened. He could now look forward, and I would help.

We scheduled Walt for a heart catheterization the next week. The findings were not surprising. The heart attack had significantly damaged his heart, leaving him with approximately 50 percent efficiency. Although a blocked artery had caused the heart attack, the other two coronary arteries had only beginning narrowing.

I discussed the findings and appropriate treatment options with Walt and Sheila. He might choose from two surgical procedures: bypass grafting to go around the blockages of his two narrowed arteries or angioplasty, which would use a balloon technique to force open the narrowings of the two arteries. There was also an appropriate and noninvasive alternative—an aggressive lifestyle management technique to slow the process of the coronary artery disease and perhaps even reverse it. After a thorough discussion, Walt opted for aggressive lifestyle management.

Together we designed a complete program for Walt. He began a slow, progressive walking program; made some dietary modifications, such as cutting down on saturated fat; and set some weight loss goals. With Sheila's support, he planned to quit smoking. In addition, I started him on a powerful cholesterol-lowering agent, one of the statin medications that have been so important in cardiovascular medicine. With all of these changes, slowly things began to turn around. After one month, Walt's endurance was better and his chest pain was less frequent. He had stopped smoking. After three months, he had lost ten pounds and felt more energetic. His chest pain continued to decrease. He had also regained his happiness and fighting spirit.

By six months, Walt's transformation was complete. He had lost twenty pounds. His total blood cholesterol level and LDL level were under control. He rarely experienced any chest pain. And he had gone back to teaching high school and coaching the football team, which filled him with pride and a sense of accomplishment. Most important, Walt had regained a sense of hope in his life. During this visit, Walt commented, "In a funny way, my heart attack was a blessing. It turned me around and helped me finally start living. I feel better, both physically and emotionally, than I have felt at any time in my life. And I now have a workable life plan to make sure I will be there to walk down the aisle with each of my daughters."

The principles of high performance health that help you prevent disease also help the healing process when you face specific health challenges.

Walt's story is by no means unique. Often, I have seen individuals, through their own efforts and with help from our research or clinical team, form a partnership that results in true healing. These individuals played an active role in the rehabilitation process, and, like Walt, most said that the process gave them not only physical benefits but a renewed sense of hope and confidence in their ability to use their improved health to achieve a better life. They truly used the power of high performance health to stimulate the healing process.

Given Walt's success, you may wonder whether it's possible to actually reverse disease. The good news is that in many cases the answer is absolutely yes. We know from many studies that individuals with significant heart disease who get their blood lipids under optimal control, start an exercise program, and participate in stress reduction can actually reverse their heart disease. If you have heart disease or risk factors for it, as many adults do, I would strongly encourage you to work with a physician who also believes in the power of the healing process. While it may be possible to achieve these positive results on your own, you will usually get the best results by working with your physician to ensure proper ongoing evaluation and to access the appropriate medical therapies often required to get your blood lipids to the low levels necessary to reverse heart disease.

Just as important, reversing the *risk* of significant illness is possible and proven. For example, we know that individuals who stop smoking reduce their risk of heart disease by half within twelve months following their last puff. We also know that patients who lose as few as five to ten pounds can often significantly reduce their need for diabetic medications or their risk of developing many of the complications associated with being overweight or obese.

HEALING WHEN YOU HAVE SPECIFIC CONDITIONS

The principles of high performance health that help you prevent disease also help the healing process when you face specific health challenges. This section explores several common medical conditions, but the principles apply to almost any health challenge.

HEART DISEASE. If you already have heart disease, the same lifestyle practices that promote high performance health can help you manage your heart disease and significantly lower your risk of having further problems. These practices include engaging in regular physical activity, getting proper nutrition, maintaining a healthy body weight, not smoking, and controlling your blood pressure. Of course, you should partner with your physician in determining what practices are right for you and in monitoring your progress as you work to strengthen your heart and prevent further damage.

If you need additional support and structure, many medical centers offer formal cardiac rehabilitation programs to support people who are recovering from a recent cardiac event and to provide long-term maintenance programs for individuals with heart disease. Usually these long-term programs are quite affordable, and participants receive monitoring not available in fitness centers.

If you'd like to learn more about using daily lifestyle practices for cardiac health, I recommend the resources available through the American Heart Association (www.americanheart.org) and the National Heart, Lung, and Blood Institute (www.nhlbi.nih.gov). My book *Heart Disease for Dummies* also provides many more details about both heart disease and the lifestyle practices I recommend.

CANCER. Many of the same lifestyle practices that help you lower your risk of heart disease can also substantially lower your risk of cancer, the second leading cause of death in the United States. Yet many people don't know this. One survey, for instance, indicated that a majority of adults felt that the risk of cancer was basically beyond their control. Yet cumulative scientific research suggests that if people would stop smoking, maintain a healthy weight, stay out of the sun during peak sun exposure, and follow a few other basic practices, we could eliminate 70 percent of all cancers in the United States.

What if you already have cancer? First, make sure you establish an ongoing and caring relationship with your primary-care doctor and the doctors taking care of your specific cancer. A supportive team approach can really help you release the healing powers of your body. In addition to working with your physician and health-care team to adopt medical and surgical therapies, research shows that many lifestyle practices, including regular exercise and proper nutrition, can play an enormous role in helping you survive or even beat cancer. As I have already indicated, a number of studies now show that becoming involved with a support group can also make an enormous difference in your survival.

The American Cancer Society provides many resources online (www.cancer.org) for information about reducing cancer risks or supporting cancer recovery. Daniel Nixon's book *The Cancer Recovery Eating Plan*[3] provides excellent information about nutritional practices for people with cancer. I also recommend the books by Bernie Siegel (*Love, Medicine and Miracles* or *Peace, Love and Healing*).[4]

OBESITY. Although 66 percent of Americans are overweight or obese, most people tend to underestimate how dangerous these conditions are. By the time a person is obese, he or she has tripled the risk of heart disease and increased the risk of diabetes by forty times. And the medical definition of obesity is not as "fat" as you may think. If you have a body mass index (BMI) of greater than 30 (roughly, that means being 30 to 40 pounds overweight), you are technically obese, and your body biologically knows it. Managing obesity isn't an appearance or acceptance issue; it's a health issue. Obesity is a major risk factor for heart disease, cancer, high blood pressure, and diabetes. Obesity has increased 40 percent in the U.S. in the last twenty years, making it the fasting-growing preventable risk factor in our country.[5]

> Managing obesity isn't an appearance or acceptance issue; it's a health issue.

If you are overweight or obese, you know that losing weight, and, perhaps even more importantly, keeping it off, can be a difficult challenge. My research organization has studied these issues for many years. In several studies, we have partnered with Weight Watchers International to test many aspects of the Weight Watchers program.

Over twenty years of research, the scientists at Rippe Lifestyle Institute have reviewed thousands of studies conducted throughout the world and have examined many of the available weight loss and weight management programs. Our goal has been to search scientifically for what works and what doesn't. What we have discovered is that the programs that work invariably incorporate the following four strategies:

A sound approach to nutrition. Eating plans include the nutrients necessary for health while reducing energy intake and increasing energy expenditure to lose weight or balancing energy intake and expenditure to maintain weight.

Regular physical activity. Getting moderate activity on most, if not all, days helps individuals maintain lean muscle and boosts metabolism and energy. Walking programs enjoy the widest appeal and success.

Adopting a long-term mind-set. Successful programs recognize that weight gain does not occur overnight and that weight loss requires a long-term strategy.

The support of other individuals. Group support helps individuals meet their weight-loss goals. This is one of the strengths of the Weight Watchers meetings. Individuals who successfully lose weight on their own often find support from their families or some other support group, such as walking partners.

Data from many studies indicate that if you incorporate these four strategies into whatever program you adopt or design, you can lose weight and keep it off. For more information about sound strategies for weight loss and maintenance, I recommend WeightWatchers.com. I have also written a book in collaboration with Weight Watchers called *Weight Loss That Lasts*,[6] which offers more in-depth information about the scientific basis for weight loss and maintenance.

HIGH BLOOD PRESSURE. More than one out of three adults in the U.S. has high blood pressure, or hypertension. That means that more than 65 million American adults suffer from this condition. High blood pressure is a major risk factor for both heart disease and stroke, so it's very important that everyone knows their blood pressure and, if it's elevated, takes action. Amazingly, however, 70 percent of the 65 million Americans with hypertension do not have their blood pressure under control![7] More education is certainly needed.

Joe Montana and I have been trying to do our part. In fact, we first met when we joined a major national high blood pressure education campaign. Joe has had high blood pressure and has successfully gotten it under control. He has also openly discussed his own experience to help people understand simple strategies that can help control their blood pressure. Many people will need to use these lifestyle strategies in conjunction with proper medication as directed by their physicians. But the combo properly applied could control almost all blood pressure problems in this country.

> High blood pressure is a major risk factor for both heart disease and stroke, so it's very important that everyone knows their blood pressure and, if it's elevated, takes action.

These lifestyle strategies include—not surprisingly—regular exercise, proper nutrition, and weight management:

- Regular exercise means simply getting involved in a walking program of thirty minutes on most, if not all, days.
- Proper nutrition means paying attention to lowering the amount of sodium (salt) in your diet, which can typically be accomplished by eating less processed foods and more natural fruits, vegetables, and grains.
- Weight management means losing weight, even five or ten pounds. If you are overweight or obese, even small weight loss will reliably help lower your blood pressure.

Joe and I have put together some powerful materials that show you how to be an active participant in helping to control your blood pressure. These can be found at our Web site, www.getbpdown.com. On the site, you can also request a free book Joe and I coauthored, titled *Joe Montana's Family Playbook for Managing High Blood Pressure.*

ARTHRITIS. More than 20 percent of all people over the age of sixty have some form of arthritis. In fact, arthritis is the leading cause of missed work days and disability in the U.S. Paying attention earlier in life to healthy lifestyle practices such as physical activity and weight management can help you avoid arthritis in later years. Paying careful attention to injury rehabilitation and healing when you have injuries to joints and surrounding tissue is also critically important.

For good general and specific information on arthritis, I recommend the Web site of the Arthritis Foundation (arthritisfoundation.org). You can also find some specific exercise programs that may help you manage arthritis in *The Joint Health Prescription*,[8] which I wrote several years ago with my team at Rippe Lifestyle Institute.

On your quest for high performance health, don't let arthritis get in your way. If you find that arthritis symptoms are interfering with your ability to carry out your physical activity program and control your weight, for example, work with your physician. Although some arthritis medications have recently been taken off the market because they were associated with some adverse side effects, including increased risk of heart disease, don't make the mistake of thinking that all arthritis medicines are dangerous. A combination of the right supportive medication and the right physical activity and weight management programs can actually help improve arthritis symptoms for most people.

SMOKING. Okay, smoking tobacco is not a disease or a health condition. But I put it in this category because it is certainly a great health risk.

And smoking can be one of the greatest barriers to achieving high performance health.

Smoking is the leading cause of preventable death in the U.S. More than four hundred thousand preventable deaths occur each year from smoking or smoking-related causes.[9] As I know from working with many patients and supporting members of my own family, it's hard to stop smoking. It's a very strong addiction. Quitting may take many tries. But the payoff for the effort and agony is worth it. Quitting smoking significantly reduces your risk of heart disease, high blood pressure, cancer, and lung disease.

> True healing, I believe, only comes from both physical and spiritual healing.

If you smoke, remember that we now have a wide range of supports available, from medication to structured programs. There are even online smoking cessation support groups. For starters, you can find resources to help you at the Web sites of the American Cancer Society (www.cancer.org), the National Cancer Institute of the National Institutes of Health (www.nci.nih.gov), the American Heart Association (www.americanheart.org), and the American Lung Association (www.lungusa.org).

I also recommend *The Last Puff*, by John Farquhar and Gene Spiller, a book that describes techniques many former smokers have used to quit the habit.[10] Please remember that your smoking harms not only you but people around you. Exposure to secondhand smoke is a very significant danger for both heart disease and cancer. Deciding to quit smoking could be the most important high performance health decision you make.

SPIRITUAL HEALING. I mentioned earlier the great importance of understanding the profound links between mind and body. If you are struggling with any of the medical conditions discussed in the previous section or with any other significant medical issue, it is important to understand the need for both spiritual and physical healing. True healing, I believe, only comes from both physical and spiritual healing.

Spiritual healing is fostered by many sources, but I recommend that you make your first priority reaching out for the support of others. This circle of support may be composed of family and friends, clergy, or individuals who suffer from the same condition you have, but the circle is important. Social isolation can inhibit healing, while social connection enhances both spiritual and physical healing.

REFRAME AND RECLAIM

Emphasizing rest and healing are two ways that you reframe lifestyle issues and health so that you can reclaim the good health that God gave you at birth. When you fail to put health problems in the perspective of health goals and life goals, you fail to take advantage of the enormous power that your body has to regenerate and repair and renew for vital living.

One of my senior executive patients struggled for years to control his weight. Each year at his health assessment, I counseled Tom that his weight was robbing him of many productive years. I urged him to think of his health as an asset to be maintained and protected just as he maintained the equipment in his plants and the well-being of his workforce. But Tom ignored the message until a major heart attack nearly killed him. That "message" reframed his perspective about what was important in his life. I'm saddened at the price he had to pay but gladdened at his turnaround. After six months of a structured cardiac rehabilitation, Tom has lost significant weight, increased his exercise, and is meditating for further stress reduction. He's looking forward to the birth of a first grandson. He has reclaimed his life and broadened his perspective about what really matters.

When it comes to stopping to heal when your body and spirit need it, I am asking you to pause now—don't wait for a major shock—

reframe your health issues, and reclaim your birthright of good health. This step is fundamental to achieving high performance health.

MAKING IT PERSONAL

Identify two specific tasks to encourage rest and healing.

Chart how you will achieve disciplined periods of rest:

Daily _____

Weekly _____

Monthly _____

List any specific health conditions that you have, and describe how you are going to reframe your actions to reclaim your good health.

_____

_____

_____

_____

8 | OVERCOME THE SEVEN MAIN BARRIERS TO HIGH PERFORMANCE HEALTH

Carpe diem! (Seize the day!)
  —LATIN PROVERB

Yeah, just sitting around waiting for my life to begin
while it was all just wasting away.
  —BRUCE SPRINGSTEEN, "BETTER DAYS"

Up to this point, I've focused primarily on the positive things you can do to turn your health into a high performance tool. It's now time to shift focus and think about some failures. We're going to explore the seven major barriers that can block your goal of achieving your best health now, and then look for ways to overcome them.

BARRIER 1: FAILURE TO FRAME ISSUES PROPERLY

This barrier is no surprise. This entire book is about reframing your health as a high performance tool rather than as the simple freedom from disease. And you've met individuals like Bill, the middle-aged school administrator who thought walking was appropriate only for his elderly parents, although he himself lacked energy, carried too many pounds, and had lost interest in life. Bill certainly was not framing his health issues as a dynamic way to get more out of life. You'll remember other examples of individuals who failed to frame their health issues in positive ways. In my experience, three types of "failure to frame" stand out as most important.

SHORT-TERM THINKING. The classic example of short-term thinking is the person who wakes up one morning, looks disgustedly at his or her pudgy shape in the mirror, and decides to go on a crash diet to lose ten pounds in the next two weeks. Of course, you may lose ten pounds in two weeks, but statistics show you're probably setting yourself up for failure. A high percentage of the weight lost in crash diets is either water or lean muscle mass, not fat. The loss of metabolically active lean muscle mass leads to a progressive slowdown in metabolism and sets the dieter up for equally quick weight regain. Virtually all the weight regained is fat, not muscle. Thus emerges the vicious cycle known as

> The key to success is to frame weight management as a long-term challenge that needs to be addressed with a long-term solution.

yo-yo dieting: each time the dieter attempts short-term weight loss, it becomes progressively more difficult to achieve. In spite of the evidence that crash diets don't work, however, our culture's desire for a quick fix is so strong that it has spawned a multibillion-dollar industry of short-term weight-loss techniques.

The root of this societywide problem in weight loss is short-term thinking. Rather than accept that effective weight loss is a slow, progressive process, many people fall prey to the misleading notion that they can solve a long-term problem with a short-term solution.

Fortunately, there is a simple solution, even if using it takes discipline, focus, and patience. Slow, progressive weight loss of about one pound per week, using portion control and regular exercise, can succeed in the long term and yield multiple health benefits. The key to success is to frame weight management as a long-term challenge that needs to be addressed with a long-term solution.

NOT TAKING PERSONAL RESPONSIBILITY FOR YOUR HEALTH. Too many people think managing their health is their doctors' responsibility. If they get sick or injured, then their doctors will write a prescription for the answer. Again, the problem has been poorly framed. Of course, medical science offers many effective drugs and procedures to assist in the maintenance of good health. However, relying on medical therapies rather than positive lifestyle practices as a frontline strategy for promoting health reflects the degree to which we have progressively "medicalized" health to be simply freedom from disease. As each of us pursues high performance health, we must recognize that the best outcome is always achieved by true partnerships between patients and physicians. Until you frame your health as primarily your own responsibility, you will have difficulty achieving the type of health that promotes the vigor and high performance we have been discussing in this book.

BELIEVING MOST DISEASE CANNOT BE PREVENTED. We have a framing problem in how many Americans view disease. For example, more than 50 percent of people feel that cancer is a matter of chance, although numerous studies have shown that over half of all cancers could be prevented if people stopped smoking, maintained a healthy weight, improved nutrition, and protected their skin from the sun's UV rays.[1] Clearly, people are not framing the problem of cancer correctly.

The same goes for taking similar lifestyle steps to reduce the epidemic of metabolic diseases in our country, including coronary artery disease, diabetes, hypertension, and many others. Not all disease can be avoided, of course, but framing the problems correctly and focusing on proven, preventive measures could help millions reduce their risks and establish a firm foundation for achieving high performance health.

BARRIER 2: ALL-OR-NONE THINKING

When it comes to changing negative health habits, many people falter by adopting an "all-or-none" approach to change. Rather than making gradual changes, they adopt a radical program and turn their lives upside down. They also use minor stumbles as an excuse to quit in their quest for better health. Such all-or-none thinking usually dooms you to failure. Change is most likely to occur if you think of it as an incremental process. Your goal is to integrate positive health behaviors gradually into your daily life.

Incremental thinking works for most tasks you undertake. For example, one regular element of my exercise routine is running four miles. I particularly enjoy running over the hilly terrain of the Berkshire Mountains. But when I first started the run, I couldn't finish the last three-quarters of a mile. The reason for this was simple. I was used to running on flat land, but this stage of my route featured climbing three progressively steeper hills to reach the plateau where our house sits. It took me about a month to figure out an effective strategy. I did this by naming each one. I named the first rise "Heartbreak Hill" after the famous set of hills at the Boston Marathon. If I could make it up the first hill, my heart would not be broken. The second hill I named "Mind-Break Hill." Making it up this hill would indicate that my focus and determination survived unbroken. The third slope I christened "Concentration-Break Hill." By the time I reached this hill, I knew that I had already climbed the two most difficult hills and that the only thing that could stop me now was to lose concentration. It may seem

> Change is most likely to occur if you think of it as an incremental process.

silly that I took the effort to name each hill, but it broke the challenging run into three smaller subgoals that made the overall task much more achievable.

You can use the same incremental approach to incorporate change into your daily life. When it comes to exercise, if you have been sedentary, start by walking one-quarter of a mile on a flat surface and slowly build up to a half mile, and so on. Use the same approach to improve your nutrition. Think about easy ways you can gradually integrate more fruits, vegetables, and whole grains into your meals and snacks.

You get my point. Don't fall prey to all-or-none thinking. Also, remember that change occurs with peaks and valleys and plateaus. Don't expect that change will be one continual progression. You will stumble and falter and even "fall off the wagon." Accept that reality, and get back on track. Don't confuse relapse with collapse. You can do better.

BARRIER 3: POOR PLANNING AND PREPARATION

Failure to plan and poor preparation are two small issues that people typically falter on when seeking changes in their health.I learned this early in my career. Many patients who started walking programs during the summer and fall in New England, for instance, had difficulty maintaining their walking programs in the winter. When they came in for their quarterly checkups in the winter, these patients had gained weight, and their fitness levels had deteriorated. When I asked why they weren't walking, they'd say, "The weather is too cold," or "I have no place to walk." As an experienced exerciser (but young physician), I hadn't thought to counsel my patients about the importance of having an all-weather warmup suit or finding an indoor environment, such as a shopping mall, to walk during the winter. These individuals didn't lack the willpower to stick to their exercise programs; they lacked the proper preparation for the change of season.

My team and I now make sure that we help patients and research participants plan and prepare properly for making important changes to achieve their health goals. Here are a few of our tried-and-true tips straight from our not-so-secret files.

- When traveling, choose hotels that have fitness centers. Even if your schedule is packed, you can get in thirty minutes on the treadmill or stationary bike.
- Wherever you go, pack your walking or running shoes. There's almost always time for a walk or jog.
- Plan an active vacation. Vacations are often more relaxing if they include sports or activities the whole family can enjoy.
- Trying to quit smoking? Avoid environments where cigarettes are readily available.

You get the idea. Spending a few minutes in planning and preparation can make the difference between success and failure.

BARRIER 4: NOT LIVING IN THE PRESENT

Many people get caught in the trap of either regretting the past or fearing the future, as I discussed earlier in the section on stress reduction. They fail to make permanent, positive change because they fail to live in and enjoy the present.

> Living in the present is not only the basis of successful stress reduction but also a recipe for enjoying life to its fullest.

I must admit I continue to struggle with this issue. At home, I am known as the family worrier because I am always planning ahead, often a bit anxiously. Stephanie has counseled me on numerous occasions that it would be better for my health and everyone else's sanity if I could focus more on the present. The roots of this issue for me, as for many people, reach back into childhood when I first began to juggle multiple tasks and goals in school and on the athletic field and beyond. Today I still wrestle with balancing the need to plan for the future with my goal of living in the present. More and more, however, I have begun to understand that having a certain level of anxiety is part of who I am, and that's okay. Accepting this aspect of myself, interestingly, helps me to focus more on the present. Of course, the most powerful impetus to live in the present is being the father of four young, engaging daughters.

Focusing on the present enables you to cope with today without carrying the emotional baggage of past regrets and future fears.

BARRIER 5: NOT RECOGNIZING THE THREE AGES WE ALL POSSESS

When it comes to our health, each of us possesses three ages:

- Chronological age: the number of years we have been on the planet
- Physiological age: the functioning age of our organs and muscles
- Spiritual age: the emotional age of our spirits

How we perceive and respond to each age can either block our efforts to achieve our best health now or encourage them.

CHRONOLOGICAL AGE. Unfortunately, our youth-obsessed culture tends to focus too much attention on chronological age, particularly on diminishing it or denying it. We spend billions of dollars trying to look younger. The many turn-back-the-clock nostrums, from beauty lotions to cosmetic surgeries, offer a very shallow appeal to appearance. The plain truth is that too many of us focus too much attention on the one aspect of age we can't change—our chronological ages.

From time to time, this is brought home to me personally. As I mentioned earlier, when my first daughter was born, I was in my late forties.

She started preschool at the age of two, and on one occasion, I went to pick her up. When she saw me, she exclaimed, "That's my daddy; he has gray hair!" Without pause, I responded, "Hart, I didn't have gray hair before you were born; what do you make of that?" (Of course, that was a fib, maybe prompted by a twinge of self-consciousness as the oldest parent there, but I also wanted to hear how she would respond.) Toddlers aren't into irony; they call it as they see it. Hart simply repeated to everyone, "That's my daddy; he has gray hair!"

She was right. Those were the facts. I am her daddy, and I do have gray hair. I think that ageless wonder and wit of baseball, Satchel Paige, would have approved of Hart. As he once observed, "Age is a case of mind over matter. If you don't mind, it don't matter."

I'm actually proud of my gray hair. I've earned it. And the perspective and maturity I've gained while earning it, I hope, make me a better father. While there are certainly times in my life that I would love to go back and fix; there are also periods that I am happy I don't have to revisit. I firmly believe that aging has multiple benefits, not the least of which is a deeper appreciation for life and a more profound ability to love.

PHYSIOLOGICAL AGE. Unlike chronological age, people can change their physiological ages by taking care of their bodies. Most people underestimate just how significant that change can be.

At Rippe Health Assessment, when we perform exercise treadmill tests, we measure the amount of oxygen an individual can consume at peak exercise. This gold standard measurement of the body's aerobic fitness shows not only the heart's ability to pump blood to exercising muscles but also the efficiency with which those muscles can extract the oxygen from the blood. We also explain to each patient how the results compare to other individuals of their age and sex. The results show that some of our patients are so fit that the aerobic capacity of their cardiovascular system far exceeds that of most individuals of the same chronological age. For example, Rick, a retired CEO of a Fortune 500 company, has an aerobic capacity greater than 150 percent of avergage for indi-viduals of his age and sex. Another patient, Phil, who will turn fifty this year and runs every morning, has a cardiovascular fitness level higher than that of the average twenty-year-old. I'm proud that my cardiovas-cular fitness level is above the average of that of a twenty-five-year-old.

These examples illustrate the power of regular physical activity to alter the physiological age of one of the body's systems. Regular exer-cise, appropriate nutrition, and other healthful lifestyle practices can create an environment for many of the body's systems in which their physiological age may be lower than their chronological age.

You might emulate a friend of mine who just turned sixty who likes to take the stairs two steps at a time and jump puddles after a rainstorm. She also likes to quote Satchel Paige when friends raise an eyebrow at these antics: "How old would you be if you didn't know how old you were?"

SPIRITUAL AGE. We all know people who are so optimistic and energetic that it is a gift to be around them. Such people seem to have discovered the spiritual fountain of youth. A sprightly African-American woman named Bea epitomizes these individuals for me. I first met Bea when she was in her eighties. She had suffered a heart attack in her late seventies and continued to experience occasional chest pain when she walked up the flight of stairs at her church. She had chosen me as a "young" car-diologist because she felt that a young doctor would have the most cur-rent information. (As I like to point out to my children, there actually was a time when I could be considered a "young" cardiologist.)

For the first few months of our consultations, I progressively adjusted Bea's cardiac medicines to try to control her chest pain. I was particu-larly concerned that she continued to climb the stairs at her church in order to teach her Sunday school class. Finally, because we were hav-ing such difficulty getting her chest pain under control, I counseled Bea that it was time for her to retire from her Sunday school class. I will never forget her response: "Dr. Rippe, I trust you to take care of my cardiac medicines and God to take care of my soul. With all due respect, teaching my Sunday school class is what keeps me alive. If I have to accept a little chest pain in order to do it, that's fine with me. When God no longer wants me to teach the Sunday school class, He'll take me away." Bea continued to teach that class for another five years and died quietly at home at the age of eighty-nine. Young doctors don't know everything, I'm glad to say. This one learned a powerful lesson in high performance thinking from Bea.

> To achieve your best health, you should avoid focusing too much on chronological age and seize the enormous opportunities to alter your physiological and spiritual ages.

Many attributes characterize people who maintain a youthful spiritual age. Perhaps the most striking feature is their willingness to take on new challenges and try new things throughout their lives. I have had patients who, after retiring from work in their seventies, started taking piano lessons, became computer experts, or adopted a new career. All found ways of interacting with other people and keeping their outlooks and spirits youthful.

If you wish to stay spiritually youthful, once again you might consider Satchel Paige's advice: "Work like you don't need the money. Love like you've never been hurt. Dance like nobody's watching."

To achieve your best health, you should avoid focusing too much on chronological age and seize the enormous opportunities to alter your physiological and spiritual ages.

BARRIER 6: FAILURE TO RECOGNIZE YOU HAVE THE POWER TO CHANGE YOUR HEALTH

When *Star Wars*' Obi Wan Kenobi counsels Luke Skywalker, "The force is within you," he might be speaking to each of us about our health. Our tendency to view good health as simply the absence of disease creates enormous problems because it bogs us down in the status quo rather than motivating us to achieve our optimum potential.

The consequences are startling. For example, a recent study by the American Cancer Society indicated that people who are obese cut their life expectancy by seven years. Individuals who smoke one pack of cigarettes per day also cut their life expectancy by seven years. Those who are obese and smoke, double their trouble, lowering their life expectancy by fourteen years.[2] Now, I don't want to minimize how difficult it is to lose weight or stop smoking. Yet each of us has the power to make those choices to improve our lives.

The evidence that you have the power to change your health is strong. The cumulative findings of hundreds of studies show that regular physical activity lowers the risk of virtually every chronic disease. When it comes to nutrition, cumulative research evidence shows that consuming five or more servings of fruits and vegetables

> The evidence that you have the power to change your health is strong.

each day and eating at least three one-ounce servings of whole grains are associated with a lower risk of many cancers as well as a lower risk of heart disease, high blood pressure, and diabetes. This list could go on and on. My point is you have the power.

BARRIER 7: THINKING THAT CHANGE IS EASY

Many people mistakenly believe that change is easy. That makes people who struggle to change feel inadequate or guilty. Everyone knows someone who says, "Quitting smoking was a snap. I just tossed out the last pack and never lit another cigarette." Or perhaps you have a coworker who loves to get up at 5:30 a.m. to walk thirty minutes in the cold and snow and then brags about it around the office coffeepot. "Losing weight is so easy," blare the radio ads. "Just take two of these pills at bedtime and sleep the excess pounds away."

But change is not easy. If you think change is easy for most but you're somehow just not getting the picture, then you've fallen for the myth of downhill running.

Which is easier—running uphill or downhill? Running downhill looks deceptively easy, but it's actually harder than running uphill (if you're a person and not a wheeled vehicle). Experienced runners know that downhill running punishes the legs because the activity asks the muscles to contract in ways they are not used to— to make "eccentric contractions," in physiological terms. The great marathoner Bill Rogers, who won the Boston Marathon many times, excelled because he was *the* master downhill runner. He could cruise down the inclines of Boston's "Heartbreak Hill" even as others crashed.

> The process of change will require your dedication and hard work.

Downhill running is a good metaphor for the subtlest barrier you face in choosing to achieve your best health now—the perception that change is easy. As a physician with more than twenty-five years' experience helping people make changes in their lives, I can assure you that change is difficult. But you can do it—you can achieve high performance health. You must recognize, however, that the process of change will require your dedication and hard work.

You may find it helpful to understand the progressive stages that most of us move through as we make the decision to change and implement our change strategies. My colleague Dr. Jim Prochaska has performed important research in this area. Here's the framework for change that he presents in his book *Changing for Good*:

STAGES OF CHANGE

I. *Precontemplation—"Get off my back."*
Others may confront you about the need to change. You may feel angry and helpless. There are constructive ways to encourage change.

II. *Contemplation—"I want to stop feeling so stuck."*
You want to change, but you're not quite ready. You can counter anxiety with excitement and knowledge.

III. *Preparation—"I'll start tomorrow."*
You know change is best, but you're not sure how to begin. Use this time to develop an effective plan of action.

IV. *Action—"Here I go!"*
Life is often exhilarating, sometimes terrifying. So is change. Learn the methods and get the support you need.

V. *Maintenance—"Keep going forward!"*
You're reaping the rewards of change, but you know relapse is common. Create a plan for dealing with slips and lapses and achieve long-term success.

VI. *Termination—"Home free!"*
Maintaining change is effortless: No temptations, total confidence. Even if you do not totally eliminate temptation (many people don't) you can still achieve lasting change.[3]

Don't let being realistic about change discourage you. Instead, understand that accepting that change is hard is an important way of giving yourself credit for your willingness to make change. You can do it. Being realistic about the challenges is the first step toward success.

MAKING IT PERSONAL
Focus on one specific change you would like to make in your life.

Write down the change you would like to make here:

_____

_____

_____

Now develop a doable strategy for overcoming the seven barriers.

How am I going to frame this issue properly?

_____

_____

How will this fit into the normal fabric of my life? (Avoid "all-or-none" thinking)

_____

_____

How will I plan and prepare to make this change?

_____

_____

What will I do starting today? (Live in the present)

_____

_____

How will this enhance my physiological and/or spiritual age?

_____

_____

How will this improve my health?

_____

_____

What will I do to make the commitment and accomplish the work to make this change a permanent part of my life?

_____

_____

9 | USE HIGH PERFORMANCE HEALTH AS A SPRINGBOARD TO HIGH PERFORMANCE LIVING

Don't be afraid of hard work or teaching your children to work.
Work is dignity and caring and the foundation of a life with meaning.
—MARIAN WRIGHT EDELMAN, *THE MEASURE OF OUR SUCCESS*

The first responsibility of a leader is to define reality.
The last is to say thank you. In between the two, the leader
must be a servant and a debtor. That sums up the progress
of an artful leader.
—MAX DEPREE, *LEADERSHIP IS AN ART*

What is high performance living? In its simplest terms, high performance living is the ability to perform at the best of your ability to meet whatever challenges are put in front of you and to do this consistently. Performing at your best means getting out of your own way and focusing on issues that make a difference to you and your loved ones. Performing at your best consistently means evaluating and responding to those issues day to day, week to week, month to month, and year to year. Whatever the challenge, the goal is doing your best based on your values, not on "winning" at all costs. Doing your best also means bringing your whole self to the job.

It has taken me a number of years, both as a physician and as a human being, to evolve this understanding of what I call high perform-

High performance living is the ability to perform at the best of your ability to meet whatever challenges are put in front of you and to do this consistently.

ance living. As a young doctor, I saw my primary job as treating physical health issues for patients. After all, physical complaints brought them to my office. It took me a while to understand that my patients' needs were much more complicated. I owe an important early insight to one of my patients, William, who had stable angina (chest pain) that we were managing. During a regular checkup, William complained that his chest pain recently had become much worse. I immediately peppered him with questions: When did the pain happen? How intense was it? What time of day did it occur? and so on. William dutifully answered all of my questions. After a few minutes, I turned to my desk to write prescriptions to adjust his medications to combat what I thought were manifestations of increased narrowing of his coronary arteries.

Once my barrage of questioning stopped, however, William said in a soft voice, "Doctor, my wife has left me." Tears welled in his eyes as he told me that after twenty-five years of marriage, his wife had decided to pursue life on her own. A moment of intense embarrassment washed over me: I had not thought to ask him what else was going on in his life. Clearly, William had come to see me not only for his chest pain but, perhaps more importantly, to receive care from a concerned friend. I put down my pen, and we talked. It was clear that his pain was more than physical, though the psychological trauma and stress of his loss were certainly contributing to his increased angina. In the end, I still adjusted his medications, but I also provided better support for William, the whole person.

All of us have times when we need the support and comfort or maybe just the listening ear of another concerned human being. On countless occasions at our clinic, in the privacy of a consulting room, outwardly cool and in-charge business executives have shared with me significant private traumas and concerns that were preventing them from living life to the fullest.

I remember Arnold, who was estranged from his oldest son. When I asked him about the quality of his emotional and spiritual life, he responded, "It has been truly said that you can never be happier than your least happy child." Despite his enormous business successes, Arnold's personal life was in shambles and his marriage was threatened because of long-standing, painful issues between him and his oldest son. During this session and over the next few years, our conversations focused on this concern. As time passed, I shared Arnold's joy that gradually he and his son were able to find a middle ground, in part by applying of some of the principles we discuss in this chapter.

There are also patients who are up-front with their broader goals. When in her midforties Mandy came for a health evaluation, unlike many patients, she already knew the wider benefits of high performance health. In the early 1980s, Mandy had been an Olympic swimmer and the fastest female freestyle sprinter in America. She had experienced high performance health. Since that time she had built a family and a business. Although she continued to exercise intermittently, she missed the fitness and pleasure she had derived from being in peak condition. She wanted once again to achieve peak conditioning, not to compete professionally in any sport but just to enjoy the health and life benefits.

> All of us have times when we need the support and comfort or maybe just the listening ear of another concerned human being.

Mandy's complete evaluation found that she was healthy and retained a high degree of lean muscle mass and aerobic fitness from her athletic background. We cleared her to resume a strenuous athletic career. A year later, Mandy was competing in triathlons, not with the goal of winning but for the sheer joy of performing at her physical best. Her business continued to thrive, and her children became her greatest supporters and cheerleaders.

Over the years, many people who have benefited from the programs of our clinic and research lab have said, "Thank you for giving me back my life." To each we say, "You took back your own life. It was our pleasure simply to provide some guidance." Personal empowerment for high performance living is the ultimate benefit of achieving high performance health.

THE PRINCIPLES OF HIGH PERFORMANCE LIVING

Anyone, whatever his current situation or challenges, can apply the principles of high performance health to an overall enhancement of living. Here are some of the most vital areas.

ENERGY. Living fully takes energy—both physical and mental energy. One of the gifts of achieving high performance health is that it provides abundant energy. The goal of high performance living is to use that energy wisely and consistently.

> One of the gifts of achieving high performance health is that it provides abundant energy.

As I have noted previously, one of the benefits of increasing your physical activity is that you increase physical and mental energy and reduce stress. The challenge, however, is how to manage that energy wisely. In *The Power of Full Engagement,* Dr. Jim Loeher and Tony Schwartz argue that one key to success is to manage energy rather than time.[1]

Where do you spend your energy? I have found that almost all the high performance athletes and executives I know have their own strategies for managing energy. Most focus on issues that are critical to their success and abandon issues that are only distractions. Spending energy on the people and activities that are important to you offers one springboard to greater fulfillment and enjoyment.

FOCUS Focus is the lens that takes the diffuse light of energy and narrows it down to the laser of performance and achievement. I have known many people who seem to have a great deal of energy but can't focus that energy on specific tasks. The ability to focus comes from practice and discipline—it's largely a learned behavior.

Consider the focus it must have taken for Joe Montana to consistently lead the champion San Francisco 49ers to more comebacks than any other quarterback and on such enormous stages as the Super Bowl. When asked how he accomplished these phenomenal results, Joe points out that the 49ers drilled over and over again on a series of plays they knew would work if everyone did their job. The team's ability to focus in the last minute of a Super Bowl came from hundreds of repetitions of simple actions, which allowed them to focus all of their energy on getting the job done in the last sixty seconds of a game.

> Breaking down big goals into smaller, specific tasks allows you to focus and helps achieve superior results.

Breaking down big goals into smaller, specific tasks allows you to focus and helps achieve superior results. This works whether you are outlining a week's activity sessions within your larger physical activity program or setting weekly goals for a three-month work project. The discipline of focus allows you to channel your energy into activities and accomplishments that are essential to high performance living.

GOAL SETTING, PLANNING, AND ORGANIZATION. Goal setting is vital to the process of high performance living, and it is the first step in the planning and organization process. Just as you set specific, achievable goals that help you achieve your fitness and health objectives, you should set goals for other areas of life. Writing down your overall goals, intermediate goals, and daily goals is one of the most important and often neglected aspects of regaining control of your life. Intermediate goals may range from one week to six months. These are goals that point toward milestones or establish deadlines. From a health perspective, it might be something like losing ten pounds over three months or establishing a regular exercise program for six months. We know from large and diverse literature that individuals who are able to establish a new behavior for six months are highly likely to retain that behavior for a lifetime. That established new behavior then enables the achievement of long-term goals. The same process applies to establishing immediate goals in various aspects of improving your overall life.

> Taking time to plan actually saves time later and can free up time for family and activities you value.

Earlier I emphasized the importance of breaking down your fitness and health plans and goals into daily tasks and writing down those tasks for each day as a management tool. The same principle applies to achieving your goals for life. Many successful executives have become experts in daily planning and organization within the framework of achieving their larger strategic and long-range plans. For example, every night before I go to bed, I try to create my next day's "project sheet" on an index card. A day planner or PDA may work for you.

Of course, taking time to plan and to create daily project sheets can be challenging, given the demands of our busy lives. But taking time to plan actually saves time later and can free up time for family and activities you value.

The first and the final parts of goal setting and planning are establishing and evaluating long-term goals. Where do I want to be five years from now? What direction do I want to pursue in my career? What are the important goals and aspirations I would like to achieve in my life? It is very difficult to move forward consistently toward improving both your health and your life unless you have a long-term vision for where you want to go.

If you wish to take away just one key message about goal setting and planning, it's this: Break your bigger tasks into small ones that can be accomplished and evaluated on a daily basis. As the Chinese proverb says, "A journey of a thousand miles starts with a single step." And here's a real-life example. I edit a major textbook on intensive care medicine that is updated every four years. The book is more than twenty-five hundred printed pages and includes contributions from more than 250 authors from diverse fields. The manuscript for this textbook is over thirty thousand typed pages. The only way for me to get this book revised and published on time is to divide the work into intermediate and daily goals for the entire four-year period. As professional planners say, we start with our end goals, and then we "back out" our intermediate and daily goals and tasks. In this way, a huge task becomes manageable and the job gets done well.

> If you commit yourself to achieving your best health, you will find that it becomes a solid platform on which you can commit yourself to broader purposes.

COMMITMENT. You can set goals and plan, but unless you commit to accomplishing them, the results will disappoint you. A business seminar speaker once drew a distinction between "commitment" and "involvement" by referring to the breakfast the group had been served. "Think about the ham-and-egg breakfast that many of you just ate," said the speaker. "In this breakfast, the pig was committed, and the chicken was involved."

Commitment means giving 100 percent of yourself. We will commit ourselves to the people and purposes we value. If you commit yourself to achieving your best health, you will find that it becomes a solid platform on which you can commit yourself to broader purposes. I opened this book by saying that we will protect what we love. Protecting ourselves and our loved ones takes commitment. Achieving our goals in life takes commitment. Giving ourselves wholly to this worthy purpose also provides joy and energy and freedom.

My ten-year-old daughter loves school and her extracurricular activities of swimming and music. On her own, she has recently begun rising each morning at 5:30. When her mother and I asked why, she excitedly said she wanted to prepare so she'd be at her best for school and her other activities. Her enthusiasm assured us that her commitment is based on joy, not fear.

When I think of commitment, I also remember Susan, a colleague at Massachusetts General Hospital, where we were both house officers in the extremely tough residency program. Susan was not only a superb physician but a concert-quality French horn player. In high school she had played first-chair horn in the American Youth Symphony, and top universities recruited her as if she were a star football player. During college, she continued to study horn with the principal horn player of a major symphony orchestra. When he discovered that she was going to medical school, however, he refused to continue teaching her—he had time only for musicians, not for doctors. His shortsighted rebuff was certainly a blow, but Susan was undeterred. She continued to play the horn all through medical school (she graduated first in her class), and even through our intense, jam-packed internships and residencies. Music nourished her soul. I remember one concert she gave during this time, playing Brahms's Horn Trio, one of the most difficult pieces for the instrument. It was a transcendent moment, lifting me out of the chaos and pressure of our work and reconnecting me to balance and order and the beauty of the human spirit. Susan was committed to the things she loved—the care of patients and the making of music—and both, I think, gave her rewards in equal measure to her commitment. Certainly, her commitment enriched those of us around her.

Committing yourself to the purposes and people you value will give back richly to your life.

PERSPECTIVE. Although I've stressed the importance of focusing on the daily tasks of improving your life, it's also valuable to step back occasionally and look at the entire process as if you were standing outside. Establishing perspective in this way helps you stay on an even keel. Having perspective is important when you hit those stretches where nothing seems to be moving forward or going your way. It's easy at those moments to bog down in the "slough of despond" or to feel stranded out "where the wild things are." Stepping back at those moments to put things in perspective helps give you the freedom to let the problems go and move forward.

> Your vision should be long-term. Keep your eyes and heart on where you want to go.

Part of gaining perspective is long-term thinking. As I noted earlier, many people falter on making lifestyle changes because they adopt quick-fix, short-term thinking. While you want to break goals into doable daily tasks, your vision should be long-term. Keep your eyes and heart on where you want to go.

Another part of establishing perspective is listening to other people and honoring their points of view. Often your friends and family can help you clarify goals or get you through tough times by giving you their perspective on a particular issue or problem.

POSITIVE HABITS AND THE PURSUIT OF EXCELLENCE. Habits are repetitive actions performed until they become so routine that we rarely think about them. Habits can be good or bad. In pursuit of your best health and life, you want to foster habits that support your goals. As Aristotle observed, "We are what we repeatedly do. Excellence, then, is not an act, but a habit." These are the sorts of habits you wish to foster.

At our clinic, we emphasize helping people either get rid of negative habits or establish positive habits. Often the process blends the two goals as individuals work to substitute positive habits for negative habits. We have found that individuals who adopt positive habits such as regular exercise or sound nutrition reap multiple benefits, not only for their health but for life in general. These practices become so ingrained that many of our patients tell me they can't conceive of a life without their regular walking program or a healthful breakfast. One goal, in both high performance health and high performance living, is to take those concepts we have discussed in the book and ingrain them so deeply in your life that they become daily habits that lead to excellence.

LEADERSHIP. I confess to being a leadership-book junkie. I own books on leadership written by authors as diverse as Norman Schwartzkopf, Rudy Giuliani, and Daniel Goleman. I like to learn from the leadership styles of different men and women. One of the books that has most impressed me is Max Depree's *Leadership Is an Art.*[2] What I find so attractive about Depree's view of leadership is his almost biblical concept that a leader establishes a "covenant" with the individuals he or she leads. To be effective, a leader not only gives direction but also serves. Even when working as a team, people give up some of their freedom and self-determination to follow the direction established by the leader. As Depree asserts, it is up to the leader, then, to cherish this gift and honor the trust of these team members and also to take their best interests to heart.

Leadership is a vastly underestimated aspect of achieving both high performance health and high performance living. Remember, you must first be the captain of your own life, and then you should lead by example in the ways you work with and relate to others. Leading may be something as simple as encouraging other family members to do their best by always doing your best. Viewing yourself as a leader helps you effectively use high performance principles, not just for your benefit but for the benefit of others around you.

RESPONSIBILITY. Part of getting the most out of your health and your life is assuming responsibility for both. Increasingly in our society, we tend to blame others for our current circumstances. Certainly, outside circumstances can affect our lives, sometimes almost overwhelmingly. We can't control those forces, but we can always take responsibility for how we respond to them. More important, much of what happens to us stems from our own choices. If you want to achieve your best health and life, you must take responsibility for your choices and actions.

I keep on my desk a quote from psychiatrist Dr. Carl Rogers that epitomizes what taking responsibility is all about: "Through accepting my own individuality which I can't expect everyone else to recognize and pat me on the back for, I shape my goals and desires. I am not compelled to be a victim of unknown forces in myself. I am not compelled to be simply a creature of others molded by their experiences or shaped by their demands."[3]

A few years ago in a media appearance for a weight-loss book I'd written, an interviewer who was also a physician said, "Dr. Rippe, your book talks about the importance of regular physical activity and proper food choices for losing weight and for keeping it off. Tell us something we don't already know. Give us something that will

> If you want to achieve your best health and life, you must take responsibility for your choices and actions.

startle people into losing weight." I told this physician what I told you earlier in the book: There is no magic solution. As long as people keep looking for some miracle, some magic that will startle them into taking action, it is highly unlikely they will lose weight and keep it off long-term.

There is no magic substitute for taking daily responsibility for your own choices and actions as you work to achieve high performance health and use it as a springboard to high performance living.

RELATIONSHIPS. The ability to establish true intimacy with others and to benefit from giving and receiving love and support is extremely important to achieving high performance living. Not surprisingly, the most successful people we encounter at our clinic routinely describe their relationships with family and friends as the most important thing to them. Supportive, valued relationships are the wind beneath their wings.

Day to day, the vital relationships I have with my wife and children give me something to live and grow for. And so often it's the small, ordinary moments that bring this home to me. Playing at writing poetry with my daughters using a refrigerator magnet set. Joining the bedtime story with all four daughters snuggled around their mother as she makes each character come alive. Cooking together with Stephanie, experimenting with the local truck farm's freshest vegetables and preparing tasty, nutritious meals to share with our four daughters. Swimming together in the early morning in a nearby college pool—just we six and the lifeguard. These small daily scenes remind me that what we love, we will protect. And what we love is worth living fully for.

> What we love is worth living fully for.

REDEFINING SUCCESS

I close this chapter by asking the question I started with: What is high performance living? In a sense, this is another way of asking how we define *success* in our lives. Your answer will differ from mine. And for both of us, the answer will continue to evolve. My measures of success as a husband and father are very different from those I had as a single adult. Measures of success for me in my fifties are very different than they were in my twenties. I no longer think that I will live forever, and I am not even sure that I want to. What I do want to do now is live fully, consciously, and meaningfully. For this reason, I strive to put into practice the principles that help me transform high performance health into high performance living. Although this journey remains a daily task and challenge, it is filled with great satisfaction and meaning. I wish for you the same journey as you make the connection between high performance health and high performance living.

MAKING IT PERSONAL

To help you convert the principles of high performance health into high performance living, this chapter's assignment asks you to do some goal setting and planning. Write down three goals and indicate how you will establish a plan and commitment to achieve these goals.

Goal #1: Short-term plan, intermediate plan, and long-term plan.

_____

_____

Goal #2: Short-term plan, intermediate plan, and long-term plan.

_____

_____

Goal #3: Short-term plan, intermediate plan, and long-term plan.

_____

_____

10 | FIND YOUR PURPOSE, AND EMBRACE YOUR DESTINY

A thought transfixed me: for the first time in my life I saw the truth as it is set into song by so many poets, proclaimed as the final wisdom by so many thinkers. The truth—that love is the ultimate and the highest goal to which man can aspire. Then I grasped the meaning of the greatest secret that human poetry and human thought and belief have to impart: The salvation of man is through love and in love. I understood how a man who has nothing left in this world may still know bliss, be it only for a brief moment, in the contemplation of his beloved.

 —VIKTOR E. FRANKL, *MAN'S SEARCH FOR MEANING*

If there were a middle ground between things and the soul
or if the sky resembled more the sea
I wouldn't have to scold
my heavy daughter.

 —JOHN BERRYMAN, *THE DREAM SONGS*

To pursue high performance health means ultimately to connect it to the things we most deeply value. This connection is the most important and, for many of us, the most difficult step. Yet it is also potentially the most rewarding part of the journey because it leads us to the well-springs of purpose and meaning.

The path to purpose and destiny continues to challenge me, but the ongoing struggle has also brought me gifts of experience and insight (some my own and some from others) that you may find helpful. If I can persuade you to join me in this pursuit and perhaps shed some light on it based on the many years that I have struggled with it myself, I will have succeeded in taking your hands in mine and helping you along the way. To that end, I offer you in this chapter a meditation on some of the qualities important for finding your purpose and embracing your destiny. It's not a "how-to" plan, because every journey is very personal.

> The final step of this journey is a voyage not only of discovery but also of rediscovery.

In many ways, the final step of this journey is a voyage not only of discovery but also of rediscovery.

QUALITIES OF HIGH PERFORMANCE LIVING

As you continue your journey toward high performance living, I invite you to join me in thinking about some of the qualities that help us build bridges to discovering or rediscovering the people, purposes, and pursuits that can give life greater meaning.

LIVING INTENTIONALLY. We always tell patients and study participants that we are not asking them to make radical changes or to turn their lives upside down. Rather, we are asking them to pay closer attention to the daily fabric of their lives. We are, in essence, asking them to live more intentionally.

Living intentionally is hard. It requires discipline. It requires stepping back and making plans and setting priorities. By discipline, I don't mean a grim denial of spontaneity and pleasure. As we have discussed, having appropriate structure in our lives helps create the flexibility and time to pursue the interests we enjoy. Intentional discipline in small things like making time for a daily walk may, amazingly, help you control the sense of chaos in other areas.

In a strange way, some of the wonderful technologies that allow us to be more productive also make daily discipline all the more important. A recent survey indicates that 40 percent of individuals do not take their earned vacation every year, and more than 70 percent of individuals work at least part of each day while they are on vacation, connected by their laptops, BlackBerries, and cell phones.[1] Now, I enjoy these modern technologies, and I am as wedded to my BlackBerry as any other traveling executive. But I also believe you need to use them intentionally, with discipline, so your life is not continually interrupted by other people's priorities.

Living intentionally also means choosing where you focus your energy and creativity. My mother gave me a vivid model for this principle in the last months of her life when I was a senior in medical school. After a four-year battle with breast cancer, she had reached the end stage. In the late 1970s, Katherine Kubler-Ross's theories about the importance of letting people talk about their fears related to dying were receiving much attention in the medical community. As an earnest medical student and son, I was determined that my mother and I would have an opportunity to fully discuss her death. After I made several attempts to get her to talk about the final stages of her cancer, my mother gently chided me, "Look, Jim, I know I'm dying. I don't want or need to talk about it. I would rather talk about the living that I am going to do for however many months I have left." That was my mother—living intentionally and high performance to the end. I smile now to think that she also had no intention of relinquishing her motherly authority to give me guidance.

LOVE AND INTIMACY. In *Man's Search for Meaning*, Viktor Frankl asserts, "Love is the ultimate and the highest goal to which man can aspire."[2]

The greatest message of human thought and belief, he feels, is that "the salvation of man is through love and in love." Dr. Frankl's conviction about love may not seem unusual unless you know that he experienced this epiphany while he was incarcerated in a Nazi concentration camp, enduring horrendous conditions and watching thousands of people sent to the gas chambers. Somehow, in the midst of the Holocaust, one of the worst tragedies in human history, Dr. Frankl managed to find consolation and affirmation in the power of love.

The poet Ezra Pound expresses a similar belief in the powerful line I shared in the opening of Chapter 1: "What thou lovest well remains, the rest is dross."

Both as a physician and as a human being, I have come to believe that love is the cornerstone of health and also an absolute essential for finding purpose and embracing your destiny. I particularly like Dr. Scott Peck's definition of love as "the will to extend one's self for the purpose of nurturing one's own or another's spiritual growth." This concept of love is deeper and more encompassing than romantic love alone. Such love provides a wellspring of meaning for life.

> Love is the cornerstone of health and also an absolute essential for finding purpose and embracing your destiny.

This love requires attention and fuels courage. It involves taking risks and making commitments. At its best, love also informs the ability to confront other people when they have fallen off the path. Love is what drives virtually everything we value. Love is the essence of how God views each of us. And God's unconditional love for us teaches us how we should view ourselves and one another.

These concepts of love have grown over time in my own life and will continue to grow. They have also made an enormous difference to me as a human being, husband, father, and physician. Until my midforties, I focused largely on professional achievements, as though somehow these would bring me the happiness and meaning I sought. Then, as I mentioned earlier, I met and fell in love with Stephanie. My relationship with Stephanie became so important to me that I feared I would lose it. I very much wanted to make her my wife but was afraid she didn't feel the same about me. When it came time to propose, I presented her with a ring on her birthday and said, "I am giving you this ring to let you know that it is my intention to someday propose marriage to you." Boy, was I nervous and scared—I couldn't even pop the question. Stephanie responded in her calm and loving way, "In my heart, I am already married to you." With that gentle encouragement, I said, "Let me start this proposal again."

We have been married now twelve years, and our love grows stronger every day. We have the normal struggles most people have, trying to find our way though a complicated world. As two very purposeful and independent people, we sometimes get in each other's way. But Stephanie's love is an anchor and a guide that enables me to be a better man, father, and physician. When I'm spinning my wheels in swampy places, Stephanie is standing on firm ground, gently pulling me out. The same is true for my children, who have taught me that there are things in this world that are more important and valuable than anything else.

In medicine, we have largely discounted the power of love. Yet without love in our lives, I believe it is impossible to find either purpose or meaning.

FAITH AND TRUST. Like love, faith and trust are also critical not only to achieving good health but to finding meaning and purpose in life. As I was beginning to write this book, my dear friend and sometimes spiritual mentor, Dr. Des Cummings, gave me *The Return of the Prodigal Son*, a book by noted theologian Henri Nouwen. I shared some of Nouwen's reflections in my discussion of hope in Chapter 6. You'll remember that Nouwen bases his meditation on Rembrandt's painting depicting the return of the prodigal son, a biblical parable. Reflecting on this painting, Nouwen thinks about what it means to be both a father and a son and considers these ideas in the context of his relation-ship to God. Nouwen also discusses what it means to come home and how "coming home" relates to faith. He writes, "Faith is the radical trust that home has always been there and always will be there."[3] *Home* in this sense is grounded in the unconditional love of God as seen in the earthly father's unconditional love for the lost son. It is not surprising to me that, in his letter to the Corinthians, the apostle Paul singles out faith with hope and love as the three keys to living an abundant life.

Having faith, not only in God's love but in yourself, is critical to developing the courage to find your purpose and embrace your destiny. Trust is equally important to this journey. Trust is the conviction that there are an order and a purpose to the world and that there is a purpose for your life if you will search for it. Trust is also a central component of love and intimacy.

> Having faith, not only in God's love but in yourself, is critical to developing the courage to find your purpose and embrace your destiny.

In my life and in my marriage, love and intimacy have grown stronger as trust has grown deeper. The "home" that will always be there for me is grounded in the unconditional love of the Creator and made real in the unconditional love of my family.

Trust and faith give me the desire and the courage to seek my best health and life.

COMPASSION. As he considers the father's acceptance of the returning prodigal son, Henri Nouwen concludes that the father's authority comes from his compassion. What a wonderful and interesting concept. The act of compassion implies that the father has not only forgiven his son but has borne some of his suffering. We as human beings, Nouwen asserts, are called upon to offer the same compassion to others that we have received from God. I have found this an enormously powerful concept in my own spiritual journey. As every parent knows, setting boundaries and disciplining children are also acts of compassion in the sense that the parent is willing to share the discomfort and sometimes emotional pain that children often experience in learning appropriate boundaries and behaviors.

Some physicians feel that they have seen so much human suffering that they have become somewhat distanced from that pain. Exactly the opposite has occurred to me. My patients' difficulties and pain affect me more deeply each year. I believe this is as it should be. Compassion joins us in community. Compassion helps us help one another. Compassion calls us out of ourselves and enables us to offer ourselves to others. These are values that give purpose and meaning to my life.

Implementing your choices for change so you can reach your health goals or life goals is not easy. Recognizing this truth about our own struggles should stir our compassion and our acceptance of the struggles of others.

ACCEPTANCE. In the opening chapter, I reminded you that you are worthy of achieving your best health and the fullest life possible. I offered you Paul Tillich's insight that the gift of grace in our lives is the understanding that we are accepted and valuable just as we are. After meditating on those aspects of himself that he finds similar to the prodigal son and those that he must develop to have the true compassion of the father, Henri Nouwen concludes that one of the biggest issues in his life is acceptance, specifically acceptance of himself. Like the prodigal son, Nouwen must accept that he is worthy of forgiveness—he is worthy of being found and loved by God.

Many of us stumble on the path to achieving high performance health and high performance living because we do not feel we deserve them. We feel guilty that our own choices and behaviors have contributed to the challenging situations we face. It's at this point that we need to accept that we are worthy of forgiveness. By acceptance, Nouwen does not mean to accept his current level of spiritual growth or even where he currently finds himself in his life. Rather, he slowly recognizes that while God has been looking for him, he has not been willing to accept that he is worthy of forgiveness. To accept forgiveness is to be able to move forward.

When it comes to finding your purpose and embracing your destiny, I don't mean to suggest that you should accept either your current health or your current level of spiritual growth. Quite the contrary, acceptance means really believing that you are worthy of the effort and the joy that come from the disciplined and thoughtful pursuit of improved health and purpose.

SPIRITUALITY. Modern medicine has often viewed spirituality as a dangerous "third rail." In electric railway systems, such as subways, the third rail supplies the high voltage that powers the train along its regular tracks. Touching the third rail means immediate electrocution. Too often in medicine, we have come to believe that if we know the signs, symptoms, causes, and pathologies of disease, we can operate on "hard facts" and avoid dealing with the nebulous qualities of the human spirit. This is a mistake. We strengthen science-based medicine when we take into account the complex nature of human life as composed of mind, body, and spirit.

> To accept forgiveness is to be able to move forward.

If you want to enhance your whole life, then you must not neglect the spirit. Spirituality can be the "third rail" in a positive sense, powering your spiritual journey just as electricity powers the train. In *The Care of the Soul*, Thomas Moore, who is a trained theologian, former monk, and practicing psychotherapist, observes that the purpose of caring for the soul is not problem solving but giving ordinary life depth and value.

By "soul," Dr. Moore does not mean an object of religious belief or immortality but something akin to what I mean by spirit. In his working definition, "soul is not a thing, but a quality or a dimension of experiencing life and ourselves. It has to do with death, value, related-ness, heart and personal substance."[4]

Although the *soul* may be difficult to define precisely, there is no question that it is related to the spiritual quality of life. And we all look for spiritual sustenance. If we would have lives rich in purpose and meaning, then our need for spiritual sustenance is as great, I believe, as our need for food.

As I look back at some of my early endeavors, which seemed random at the time, I realize many of them were efforts to find and shape the spiritual quality of my life and my soul. As an undergraduate, I immersed myself in trying to become a writer. A rare opportunity to study with the great American poet Robert Lowell ultimately convinced me that I had neither the passion nor the tal-

> If you want to enhance your whole life, then you must not neglect the spirit.

ent to become a poet. But the urge to create gave me vitality. Between college and medical school, I worked several years as a studio potter making ceramics and briefly as a chef. Until my midtwenties, I had no idea my true vocation was to be a physician. Yet these seemingly random activities nurtured my spiritual life, helped define me as a person, and ultimately helped make me a better physician—one who is passionate about nurturing the whole person in medical practice and passionate about continuing to grow.

Today the creative and the artistic continue to complement my scientific life. My wife and I devote enormous energy to gardening and landscaping. We fill our work and living spaces with beautiful orchids. We often read poetry to each other and cherish those times when we can cook and create new dishes together. I tell you this because I believe these activities, some of which I simply stumbled upon, nurture my own spiritual life and feed my soul.

As you pursue high performance health and use its power in your journey to find purpose and meaning, I urge you to pay close attention to spiritual activities that feed the soul. Experiment. Pursue your passions and dreams. Make your own discoveries. You must nourish your spirit and soul if you wish to find purpose and fulfillment.

JOY. Joy is closely linked to meaning in life. By joy I do not mean the transient quality of pleasure. Rather, I mean the deep-seated sense of well-being that comes from finding fulfillment and meaning in life. It must have been joy that Ezra Pound experienced toward the end of his magnificent work, *The Cantos,* when he exclaimed, "What splendor it all coheres." As Henri Nouwen considers some of the issues that have prevented us from finding this sense of coherence, he concludes, "Joy and resentment cannot coexist." So there may be some burdens you need to lay down in order to open the door to joy.

> Joy has great power to give meaning. Open yourself to being surprised by joy.

You may also need to practice living in the present. As the family worrier, I sometimes spend so much effort planning how to smooth the paths for my family and keep them secure that I miss the joys of the moment. Stephanie continually has to pull me back into the present and remind me to stop and experience the joy of simply being with our daughters as they grow into beautiful young women.

Each of us will find our own path to joy. What's important to remember is that joy has great power to give meaning. Open yourself to being surprised by joy.

GRACE. Perhaps you first encountered the concept of grace as I did in the recordings of "Amazing Grace" by Guthrie and Baez and other folk singers. Many of us boomers thought this hymn was a folk song, but these famous words by John Newton date back to the eighteenth century.

Amazing grace! How sweet the sound
that saved a wretch like me!

I once was lost, but now am found,
was blind, but now I see.

'Twas grace that taught my heart to fear'
and grace my fears relieved.
How precious did that grace appear
the hour I first believed!

Through many dangers, toils, and snares,
I have already come;
'tis grace hath brought me safe thus far,
and grace will lead me home.

It has always struck me that John Newton immediately recognizes grace as "amazing." He recognizes grace as a gift of acceptance waiting for us to see and receive. In Scott Peck's view, grace is a powerful force outside ourselves that nurtures spiritual growth. For me, grace in one sense is the collective unconscious that empowers us to do good. Grace is available to all but also individual. Over hundreds of years, Newton's words continue to touch us with power, because they are so personal. Here is a man who has been freed from fear and filled with praise and joy by grace. We can identify.

I have often thought that our modern lives would be far better off if we allowed our lives to be permeated with grace. We often speak about "grace under pressure" or "grace under difficult circumstances." This kind of grace implies a freedom from the fears about oneself that allows one to act with power. Again, you will need to discover for yourself how grace works in your life, but seeking and accepting its amazing power will open your life to greater purpose and achievement in your every endeavor.

GROWTH AND MATURITY. Essential to finding purpose and meaning in life is having the courage to grow and mature. Growth can be painful, but you can't go forward without it. I've shared many examples in this book from my experience as a parent, in part because to help our children grow and mature, we parents must continue to grow and mature. But venturing into the unknown can be scary. Here other values we've discussed, such as courage, faith, and trust, can come to your assistance.

A friend of mine once shared with me a metaphor for change he found encouraging as he faced the challenges of becoming a university president: "Change is always difficult, but I view it as if I were a trapeze artist. The only way I can complete my trick in midair and land safely is if I have absolute confidence that, as I spin through the air having left one trapeze, there is another trapeze swinging in my direction." What a wonderful definition of growth and maturity. We can only leave our current situation if we have the absolute courage and conviction that another trapeze is swinging in our direction. (Goal setting and planning, I might note, can help you have faith in that trapeze.)

ALONENESS VERSUS LONELINESS. Although many issues related to pursuing purpose and meaning will involve the support of other people, some aspects are deeply personal. To accomplish these goals, you will need to be alone but not lonely, an important distinction that Scott Peck draws. I bring this to your attention to remind you that while you will need to grapple with many issues in quiet communication with your thoughts and spirit, you should not feel isolated or deserted. Part of the path toward finding meaning and purpose in life is accepting that a portion of this journey must necessarily occur alone.

TELLING YOUR STORY. Human beings pass down much wisdom from generation to generation through storytelling. One of the great privileges of being a physician is that I get to hear other people's stories and learn and grow from what they tell me. I've shared many stories in this book drawn from the experiences of many people. As one senior executive likes to remind us, "Every leader is telling a story about what he or she values."

Not only can we learn from the stories of others, but each of us has a story to share. A valuable part of creating purpose and meaning in your life comes from sharing your story. Your example and your wisdom, giving of yourself, can touch and inspire other people in ways you may not imagine.

FINDING YOUR PURPOSE AND EMBRACING YOUR DESTINY

Much of this chapter has focused on those aspects of life I am convinced are essential not only to good health but to the broader issues of finding purpose and meaning in life. While much of the discussion focused on qualities or activities that help us find our purpose and meaning, I am also left with the inescapable feeling in my life that there is a higher power that ultimately provides meaning and purpose to all of life.

> A valuable part of creating purpose and meaning in your life comes from sharing your story.

I encourage you to look within to discover the part of God that dwells inside each of us and the empowerment that provides. Look within to identify those values and qualities that move you forward. Look without to see how and where you can grow and contribute. In everything, I encourage you to think and live intentionally.

In the final analysis, the same discipline and courage that are required to change your health from the passive freedom from disease to a high performance tool are the same traits that allow you to accomplish the even more satisfying process of finding your purpose and embracing your destiny—of excelling at high performance living. As the narrator of Marilynne Robinson's *Gilead* says, "Precious things have been put into our hands and to do nothing to honor them is to do great harm."[5] Your health and your life are precious gifts. My deepest wish is for you to have the courage and discipline to honor them.

MAKING IT PERSONAL

In Chapter 9's assignment, you identified three goals you wished to achieve and outlined specific plans to achieve them. For each goal, decide which values or qualities discussed in this chapter can help you achieve the goal.

Goal #1:

_____

_____

Goal #2:

_____

_____

Goal #3:

_____

_____

PART 2 | ACTION PLAN

11 | TEN STEPS TO ACHIEVING HIGH PERFORMANCE HEALTH

And what there is to conquer
By strength and submission, has already been discovered
Once or twice, or several times, by men whom one cannot hope
To emulate—but there is no competition—
There is only the fight to recover what has been lost
And found and lost again and again, and now, under conditions
That seem unpropitious. But perhaps neither gain nor loss.
For us, there is only the trying. The rest is not our business.

   —T. S. ELIOT, "EAST COKER," *THE FOUR QUARTETS*

I never told you it would be easy,
I only told you it would be worth it.

   —VINCE LOMBARDI

This chapter provides a framework of ten steps that provide structure to support your pursuit of high performance health. These steps encapsulate key points I've presented throughout the book. My goal is to help you implement each step by providing a brief rationale and how-to guidance for each step. I will also discuss how you can integrate many of the steps as you implement them.

While ten steps may seem daunting, you aren't going to tackle them all at once. And if you have been doing the assignments at the end of each chapter, you have already begun incorporating them into your daily life. I recommend that you take one step at a time, perhaps one a week for ten weeks. You need not even start with step 1 but may pick another that better fits your needs and goals. Remember, too, that lasting change results from breaking larger goals into simple, achievable steps. The specific tips and suggestions may help you there.

> The ten steps to achieving high performance health are designed to help you bring health into the circle of values that undergird your life.

As you think about these ten steps, remember that the overall goal is to tie your health to your value system. What you love, you will protect. The ten steps to achieving high performance health are designed to help you bring health into the circle of values that undergird your life. In this way, achieving your best health can become a high performance tool that helps you reenergize your whole life.

To assist you, we are working on a companion workbook that will provide additional structure and guidance and a means to record your progress as you move forward on the path toward high performance health.

STEP 1: ASSESS YOUR HEALTH, SET YOUR GOALS, THEN TRACK THEM

Too many people live as if life were a game of chance. They believe there is little they can do to affect the course of their future, so they don't even try. High performance health individuals, on the other hand, take time to critically analyze their direction for their health and their lives. Then they take action toward their destination. No matter what your life dreams, you will not achieve them without a plan. Of course, it is unrealistic to think that you can control every aspect of your life. You can't. But as the old adage cautions, "If you don't know where you're going, you will probably end up somewhere else." A life without direction is a life without purpose or discipline. Examining your direction in health is an important first step.

"Robert" had not thought seriously about his health's direction before he came to our clinic for an evaluation. He'd been too busy managing and building his company. Robert was a senior executive for a Fortune 500 company. When he weighed in, the scales stopped at 320 pounds. For years, various physicians had told him he needed to lose weight. But he ignored them and got on with his work.

When I first met Robert, I asked him, "How would you rate your health?" He responded, "I'm basically healthy, but I'm too damn fat!"

"Robert," I said, "there is no question that you are significantly overweight, but before you leave our clinic today, you will recognize that you cannot use the words 'healthy' and 'too fat' in the same sentence."

We put Robert through a series of tests and found that his weight was causing a ripple effect throughout almost every metabolic system of his body. He had the beginnings of diabetes, high blood pressure, and a cluster of abnormalities called "the metabolic syndrome," a significant risk factor for coronary heart disease. Moreover, a high-speed CT scan of his coronary arteries revealed the beginnings of significant arthrosclerosis (the process of narrowing of the coronary arteries) in all three arteries supplying his heart.

> No matter what your life dreams, you will not achieve them without a plan.

When I met with Robert at the end of the day, I said, "I know that doctors have been telling you for many years that you need to lose weight. What they probably didn't tell you is that if you do not lose weight, it is unlikely that you will be alive five years from now. Even if you are alive, you are facing years of misery from diabetes and heart disease. All of the hard work you have put into establishing your career could go down the drain unless you pay attention to your weight."

It was a sobering discussion, but Robert took the advice to heart. He took stock of what he valued about his life and resolved to take control of his health by adopting lifestyle strategies that would help lower the health risks associated with the metabolic syndrome. Our nutrition team gave him a personal digital assistant with software to help him determine exactly what he was eating and to keep track of all foods and their composition, including the amount of fat and calories. And he undertook a gradually increasing program of moderate physical activity. To his credit, Robert applied the same discipline to turning around his weight and health that he had used to become successful in his business career.

A year later, when I saw Robert in the clinic, he had lost 120 pounds! With tears in his eyes, he said, "Thank you for giving me back my life." I responded, "Robert, you gave yourself back your life. Last year, I saw two of you. What you did over the past year is get rid of one of you—the 'you' that was destroying your health." I am pleased to tell you that Robert's tests that day showed his diabetes and hypertension had gone away. His lipid profile had dramatically improved, and his fitness level had doubled. He was well on his way to achieving the health that he deserved.

> If you want to achieve high performance health, I strongly recommend that you track your goals and record them on a daily, weekly, and monthly basis.

Of equal importance, Robert had discovered an unexpected reservoir of energy. Now, five years later, Robert has kept the weight off and is continuing to reap the benefits of high performance health.

Whether you face severe health challenges like Robert or not, his success demonstrates the power we have over our own health and the importance of keeping track of our progress. Once Robert got the message about the power that he had over his own health, he began to keep track of his personal habits with a PDA and became so devoted to it that he kept it with him at all times.

If you want to achieve high performance health, I strongly recommend that you track your goals and record them on a daily, weekly, and monthly basis. You may choose to use a PDA like Robert did, or you may use a day planner or journal. Keeping track of your specific steps on the road to high performance health helps you establish the discipline and structure needed to launch this process.

TIPS:

- Obtain a PDA, planner, or journal and begin writing your goals for each day. Also track the steps you take toward those goals.
- Record your weekly goals at the beginning of each week and your monthly goals at the beginning of each month. Assess your progress toward those goals each week and month.
- Consider obtaining the *High Performance Health Workbook* to use as a study guide and record keeper along with this book.

STEP 2: CONNECT WITH YOUR BODY AND MIND

In Chapters 2 and 3, I discussed the importance of tapping into your body-mind-spirit connections to achieve high performance health. This is key to mastering the mind-set. Many high performance athletes and high-level business executives have reported that how they frame issues accounts for at least 50 percent of their success. As one Fortune 500 CEO said to me, "At the highest levels of corporate America, everybody is talented. The difference between those who succeed at the very highest levels and those who do not is usually their mental focus and emotional strength."

There is no question that thoughts and feelings affect performance. For example, in my research laboratory, we conducted a study exploring mind-body links during a walking program. One group of participants simply walked thirty minutes a day. The other group combined a walking program with a simple meditation based on Herb Benson's classic *Relaxation Response*. We told these individuals to develop a phrase to repeat over and over during their walk. Some people used the phrase "left, right, left, right" in sync with each step. Some used the phrase "one, two, one, two." Still others repeated a short meaningful phrase.

At the end of twelve weeks, participants in both groups had improved their fitness levels. However, the group who added a meditative mental strategy to their walking also achieved significantly more stress reduction and improvement in quality of life compared to the individuals who simply walked. Although this experiment may seem simple, it demonstrates how powerful the links between mind and body can be.

There are many effective techniques for tapping into the mind-body link. These may include positive self-talk, concentration enhancement, biofeedback, and mental imagery rehearsal. Let me give you another example. Our research lab conducted a study of participants who were experiencing significant stress. Individual participants wore heart rate monitors and were seated in a quiet room. We asked

There is no question that thoughts and feelings affect performance.

them to focus consciously on slowing their heart rate by repeating the phrase "down, down, down" in a soft voice while concentrating on lowering their heart rate. If other thoughts came into their mind, we told them not to judge those thoughts but simply to let them go and repeat the cadence "down, down, down." During this four-week experiment, individuals who learned how to focus on the simple physiologic parameter of their heart rate were able to lower their blood pressure, decrease their stress level, and lower their heart rate. This result will not come as news to anybody who has studied the practices of the Tibetan monks, who are able to lower their heart rate to phenomenally low levels simply through their meditation.

As with this study, many other studies show that very simple bio-feedback devices, such as a heart rate monitor, can help people tap into the power of the mind-body connection. Even something as simple as paying attention to your breathing can make an enormous difference. This technique of focused breathing, for instance, is used in both yoga meditations and karate. One technique for enhancing performance in karate uses breathing to center the practitioner in the here and now. The Japanese word for this technique literally means "no mindedness." This concept doesn't mean that you are not thinking but that you are totally alert and connected to your own mind. This state removes fear and misperceptions that interfere with the execution of advanced karate movements.

I encourage you to explore various techniques and ideas that help you draw on the power of the mind-body-spirit connection.

TIPS:
- Purchase a heart rate monitor and practice calmly slowing your heart rate by repeating the phrase, "down, down, down."
- Develop a meditative phrase you can use during your walking or jogging routine. It may be as simple as "left, right" or "one, two."
- Visualize success during times of high stress. Use positive self-talk to increase your likelihood of succeeding.
- Join a yoga or tai chi class. Be sure to pick a class or style of the art that fits your current fitness level and your interests.

STEP 3: USE THE ACTIVE REST PRINCIPLES

Rest may be the most underestimated facet of high performance health. In our fast-paced society, we constantly strive to do more each day in our work, play, or entertainment. In Chapter 7, I discussed the importance of a good night's rest. Adequate rest and sleep are vital building blocks for achieving high performance health. Many people do not recognize that rest is actually a very dynamic process that gives the body and the mind an opportunity to accomplish the vital repair and maintenance work that keeps us healthy, both physically and mentally. Beyond getting a good night's sleep, I recommend three levels of disciplined rest.

> Adequate rest and sleep are vital building blocks for achieving high performance health.

Level 1: Day breaks. Take many short rest breaks of five to ten minutes during the busy day to center yourself and provide a mental respite.

Level 2: Weekly rest. Set aside one day each week (or at least a half day) to step away from work and restore balance to your physical, mental, spiritual, and social life. This wise practice forms part of virtually every major faith tradition, although you need not be religious to take advantage of its benefits. Sadly, many of us have gotten away from observing the Sabbath as a day of rest not only for our physical bodies but for our minds and spirits.

Level 3: Personal retreat. Plan a vacation or a weekend retreat on a regular basis. You may choose a peaceful location or an active location that fosters a peaceful frame of mind. You goal is to rejuvenate your spirit by getting away from the rush and demands of most modern lifestyles.

TIPS:

- Set aside several occasions during the day for breaks. Write these in your calendar specifically as "day break #1" and "day break #2." Don't let other activities intrude upon these breaks.
- Establish the discipline to set aside one day a week to rest and restore balance to your mental, physical, and spiritual life. For many people, this will be the Sabbath.
- Begin to plan personal retreats on weekends or even a weeklong vacation. Establish the discipline to plan vacations as times to rejuvenate your mind and spirit.

STEP 4: ESTABLISH A THIRD PLACE

Most people have two places where they spend a majority of their life—a work place and a home place. Each of us also needs a "third place" in which to thrive. A third place is a spot where you can go and be with like-minded people or participate in activities that refresh, reaffirm, and validate you through a shared interest or goal.

A third place may be a spiritual group, a hobby guild, an educational group, a health club, or a charity association, for example. Typically, it's a group of people who share your passion for and interest in a given activity or cause. Being active in this third place brings joy and affirmation and bolsters emotional and social health.

Recently, more people have begun to ask if virtual communities on the Internet, such as interest groups, chat rooms, or even gaming groups, can serve as third places. I think it may be too soon to say for sure. My concern is that Americans over the last decade report a decrease in the number of close friends or family in whom they can confide. Online communities may give the appearance of connection without providing the full benefits of relating to people face-to-face. My advice would be to enjoy virtual communities but avoid substituting them for face-to-face communities.

TIPS:

- Establish a "third place" and make a concerted effort to participate on at least a weekly basis. Options might include:
  - Place of worship
  - Social or educational club
  - Volunteer organization
  - Health club
  - Sports team
  - Reading group or book club
  - Hobby club

STEP 5: SET ASIDE FIFTEEN MINUTES OF SOLITUDE

As Henry David Thoreau famously observed, "Most men lead lives of quiet desperation." In our increasingly fast-paced world, most of us never take time to experience the benefits of solitude. This can lead to lives that feel wildly out of balance.

Although being connected to other people is very important (it's step 9 and relates to step 4), each of us needs time apart by ourselves. To paraphrase Walt Whitman, we need to be able to loaf and invite our souls. How else will we get comfortable in our own skin?

In my own journey in interpersonal relationships, I had to take time to be alone and come to know and nurture my own spirit before I could truly embrace the marriage and family life I cherish so much now. I am convinced that many people clutter up their lives and don't take time to be alone because they are afraid of what they might find. You cannot achieve your best health, however, until you come to know yourself.

No matter how busy you are, I strongly recommend establishing fifteen minutes each day to seek solitude. The only requirements are that you remove other distractions and be quiet. This solitude can take many different forms, including listening to music, reading a book, going for a walk or a jog, or simply sitting quietly, thinking your own thoughts. I know of one woman, a remarkable leader well into her eighties, who, wherever she was in the world and whatever the demands on her time, always set her alarm fifteen minutes before she needed to arise and spent that time in meditation and prayer. As you know, I like to jog or swim, tuned to my own thoughts.

> Although being connected to other people is very important . . . each of us needs time apart by ourselves.

Stephanie and I have found that solitude is also important for our children. It is during such times alone that children begin to build their imaginations, dream big dreams, and develop an inner life by becoming comfortable with themselves. In their classic book *The House of Make-Believe*, Dorothy and Jerome Singer argue that our excessive use of television, often as a babysitter, robs children of the opportunity to develop an inner life by providing so much overload that the child never experiences the joy of being alone with his or her own thoughts.[1] Most adults also have difficulty with this fundamental concept of being alone. Coming to terms with your inner life, however, is a vital step toward achieving high performance health.

TIPS:

- Develop the discipline of finding fifteen minutes of solitude each day. Make this a specific appointment in your daily schedule by marking it as "personal time." Identify several activities that you might like to do during this time. These could range from a time of reading and meditation to outdoor activities such as walking or gardening.
- Consider making one of your weekly retreats (step 3) a time of intentional solitude.

STEP 6: ENGAGE IN THIRTY MINUTES OF PHYSICAL ACTIVITY

The closest thing we have in medicine to a "magic bullet" is regular physical activity. But most Americans are sedentary. By getting the recommended levels of regular physical activity, you can lower your risk of heart disease, high blood pressure, diabetes, some cancers, and other chronic diseases. You will also reduce stress and increase energy. These benefits certainly foster high performance health.

How much physical activity is enough? The science-based physical activity guidelines for adults recommend that you accumulate thirty minutes of moderate intensity physical activity on most, if not all, days. The key words in this recommendation are *accumulate* and *moderate*. *Accumulate* means looking for the nooks and crannies in your daily life when you can be active. From walking after lunch to climbing the stairs to raking a few leaves, the minutes can mount up. *Moderate* means moving at a pace that lets your body know it is working, but not so intensely as to make you short of breath or unable to carry on a conversation.

If you have been sedentary, getting thirty minutes of physical activity daily may seem daunting. However, it's okay to start slowly. Getting outside to walk just five to ten minutes will begin to show you benefits, and you can build up to thirty minutes over a period of time.

As a final boon, physical activity enables you to accomplish several steps toward high performance health simultaneously. Your thirty minutes of physical activity can also count as your fifteen minutes of solitude, step 5. As you develop confidence in your routine, you can also start to add mental strategies, thereby combining it with step 2.

TIPS:

- Commit to starting a program of regular physical activity. If you have been sedentary, start with five or ten minutes of walking and slowly increase to thirty minutes on most, if not all, days. Our walking program in the appendix gives you a schedule.
- Purchase appropriate equipment before you start. For walking, you will need a pair of good walking shoes and perhaps an all-weather exercise outfit.
- Keep your activity program simple. For more than 90 percent of people, regular walking offers the right level of physical activity. You can vary your walking program with indoor or outdoor cycling, swimming, or any other accessible moderate activity.

STEP 7: DISCOVER YOUR SPIRITUAL AGE AND LIVE IT

In Chapter 8, we discussed the three "ages" each of us has. The first age is your chronological age. This reflects the number of years you have been on the planet. The second age is your physiological age. This reflects how well you have taken care of yourself. The third age is your spiritual age. This is the age with which your mind and spirit approach the world each day.

Your chronological age is a fact. Nothing you do can change it, although in our youth-obsessed culture, many people spend incredible energy and resources trying to look younger than they really are.

You can, however, do a lot to affect your physiological age. By working to achieve high performance health, you can lower your physiological age for many of your body's systems. Patients in our clinic have lowered their physiological ages by 20 to 30 percent, based on healthful activities that they have performed over the course of the year. You can do the same.

Yet when it comes to our spiritual age, most of us do not spend enough time nurturing this vital aspect of our health and well-being. We all know individuals who are so intellectually curious and spiritually alive that they seem much younger than their chronological ages.

When I think of intellectual and spiritual age, I remember my friend and mentor Dr. Ed Budnitz, who was a senior faculty member at the University of Massachusetts Medical School when I joined the cardiology department. In his mideighties and vigorous, "Bud" remained involved in patient care and as sharp as a tack. When people asked him when he was going to retire, he always responded, "I enjoy what I do so much, I see no reason to retire. Retirement is something for old folks!" When we did a walking study to establish fitness norms for people between the ages of twenty and seventy, Bud chided me for ignoring people in their eighties when it came to fitness walking. He was ready to volunteer. Bud continued to serve on the faculty the entire time I was at the University of Massachusetts and ultimately lived until his midnineties.

Following Dr. "Bud's" example, I often advise patients to work as long as they can or make specific plans to have an active and intellectually stimulating retirement. Retiring to "take it easy" can be a slippery slope to decline.

A youthful spirit, I caution, doesn't mean a childlike spirit. Experience and years bring perspective, richness, and wisdom. A youthful spirit, for me, means staying alert and eager for the possibilities of exploration, growth, and new ideas. Individuals who seek new spiritual and intellectual challenges and pick up new activities tend to retain higher levels of vigor

> We nurture those things we value, so it is important to make the effort to nurture your spirit.

and intellectual capacity than those who do not. Physical activity also promotes better cognitive function.

The first step to enhancing your spiritual age is to recognize that this is an important component of health and meaning. We nurture those things we value, so it is important to make the effort to nurture your spirit. Chapter 10 provides additional thoughts on this issue.

TIPS:

- Nourish your spiritual age by participating in your place of worship or faith community, engaging in meaningful group studies, or taking courses in spiritual subjects that interest you.
- Stimulate your lifelong intellectual capacity by doing puzzles such as crosswords or sudoku, joining a book club, taking up a new hobby, or continuing your education at a college or university or through self-directed study.
- Stay physically active to improve cognitive function.
- Cultivate a positive, upbeat outlook on life.

STEP 8: EAT TO FUEL PERFORMANCE

What we eat clearly contributes to our health. In fact, seven out of the twelve leading causes of death in the United States have a nutrition- or alcohol-related component. As the body's primary source of energy, food has the capability of either fueling or fatiguing your daily performance. In Chapter 3, we discussed the basics of good nutrition for healthy weight management.

When it comes to nutrition, we have almost too much information available. We are bombarded daily with hype for the latest "miracle" foods or diet. Each promises nutritional nirvana by "enlightening" us to some "new" food or eating pattern that will solve all of our nutritional problems.

Obviously, good nutrition is not that easy. However, both my clinic and my research organization have been actively involved in researching nutrition and performance for many years. We have developed brief guidelines anyone can follow. These basics support your efforts to achieve better nutrition, weight management, and daily energy to fuel high performance health.

Eat breakfast. Highly respected writer for the *New York Times* Jane Brody was once asked what was the most important nutritional concept she had learned in twenty-five years of writing about nutrition and health. She responded, "It's simple: breakfast like a king, lunch like a prince, and sup like a pauper."[2] This is excellent advice—you should match your calorie consumption to your calorie needs.

Your body needs calories to start the day. Eating breakfast enhances your metabolism and helps you control how much you eat later in the day. A majority of studies also indicate that individuals who eat a healthful breakfast are likely to better manage their weight. Plus, many of the foods that we enjoy regularly at breakfast, such as whole grain cereals, fruit, juice, and nonfat milk, not only fuel energy and performance but also fight disease. Consuming a low-fat, healthy breakfast is perhaps the most important single piece of nutritional advice I can give you.

Consume more fresh fruits, vegetables, and whole grains. Most surveys show that fewer than 25 percent of American adults consume the recommended five servings of fruits and vegetables daily. What a missed opportunity. Fruits, vegetables, and whole grains provide rich sources of the antioxidants, vitamins, and phytochemicals (plant chemicals) that are so important for good health. They are also loaded with complex carbohydrates that promote the slow and consistent release of energy throughout the day. Moreover, we have learned that eating the actual fruits, vegetables, and whole grains works much better than taking supplements when it comes to health and nutrition benefits.

Eat less salt. The average American adult eats five times as much salt as recommended by the American Heart Association. This habit contributes to the alarming prevalence of high blood pressure in the U.S. One of the first things Joe Montana did when he discovered that he had high blood pressure was to follow his doctor's advice to remove the saltshaker from the table and not add extra salt to foods. Unfortunately, much of the salt we consume is hidden in processed foods. By eating more fresh fruits and vegetables and whole grains, you automatically reduce the amount of salt in your diet.

Eat more fish. Fish provides an excellent source of high-quality, low-fat protein. The American Heart Association recommends the consumption of at least two fish meals weekly. In our family, we consume at least four servings of fish every week. Of course, we are blessed to be on the East Coast, where fresh fish is readily available. One word of caution: Be careful about the preparation. You can easily turn fish into a high-fat meal by frying it or covering it with bread crumbs and oil. We always grill our fish. When it comes to preparing fish, keep it simple! (If you have concern about contaminants in fish, consult the latest fish consumption advisories for your area by going to www.usasearch.gov and entering "fish consumption advisories" in the search window. The latest studies indicate that the benefits of eating fish far outweigh the possible dangers.)

> Proper nutrition can be a great tool for health and performance.

Consume less fat. The average American adult consumes too much saturated fat, which contributes to elevated cholesterol. As a cardiologist, I am concerned about the popularity of so-called low-carb diets, which in reality are high-fat diets. Both of the most popular low-carb diets of recent years derive about 60 percent of calories from fat. I have seen too many patients come in with their cholesterol greatly out of control while trying to lose weight on these diets. Every major nutritional organization recommends decreasing the amount of fat in our diet, particularly saturated fat and trans fat. I recommend that you consume no more than 20 to 25 percent of your calories in fat, and most of those fat calories should be monounsaturated or polyunsaturated.

Drink plenty of water. Water is more vital to the body's functioning than food. Even mild dehydration can cause fatigue or difficulty concentrating. So you need to be sure to drink adequate water, as I explained in Chapter 3. We get water from the foods we eat and from all beverages, but drinking plenty of pure water is a high performance goal.

Proper nutrition can be a great tool for health and performance. Here are a few summary tips.

TIPS:
- Eat a low-fat breakfast every day. I recommend a bowl of whole-grain cereal, an 8-ounce glass of juice, a piece of fruit, and coffee or tea if you enjoy these beverages. You may also enjoy nonfat milk. This low-fat breakfast will provide half the recommended daily servings of whole grains and fruits before you even take off your pajamas!
- Consume at least one fruit and one vegetable with every meal. Pick fruits that are in season. Make sure that you always have fresh fruits available in your house.
- Eat at least two servings of fish every week. Use a low-fat method of preparation, such as grilling.
- Drink plenty of water. Keep water handy during work and recreation.

STEP 9: CONNECT WITH OTHERS

True connection with others is a vital part of achieving high perform-ance health and provides joy and meaning. By connectedness, I don't mean simply being with other people, but communicating and relating at deeper levels. That takes discipline.

Not only will these connections increase the joy in your life, but a growing body of research also suggests that loving relationships improve your long-term health. Among the benefits are lowered risk of heart dis-ease, lower blood pressure, improved ability to withstand stress, improved immune function, and a slower progression of disability in age-related conditions such as arthritis.

> A growing body of research also suggests that loving relationships improve your long-term health.

The first component of establishing connections to others is to recognize their value. In our fast-paced, success-oriented world, we tend to place a higher value on achievements than on interpersonal relationships. Yet in my clinical experience, most of the people who have achieved the highest levels of both health and success also have strong connections with other human beings.

The cornerstones of connecting to others are trust and love. I have discussed these traits in great detail in Chapter 10.

TIPS:

- Take specific steps each day to nurture relationships with those around you, and show them the value you place on their friendship.
- Spend time with people you value.
- Plan specific activities you can do together with the most important people in your life.
- Do whatever is necessary to stay connected with important friends despite distance, such as e-mailing, phoning, or visiting.

Don't let important relationships lose steam becauseof distance.

- Look for ways to invest in other people so they will experience your love, compassion, and respect.
- Recognize that nurturing relationships requires commitment.

STEP 10: CONNECT WITH YOUR SPIRIT

Connecting with your spirit involves recognizing that you are more than the sum of your physical parts. There is a spiritual center to life. Each of us is designed to enjoy a personal relationship with our Creator and to recognize that there is a divine purpose to life. Whether or not you frame this step as a religious issue, it is important to regularly touch and nurture your emotional and spiritual core. The disciplined process of connecting with your spirit is vital to adding meaning, hope, comfort, and peace to life.

I must admit I don't have any final answers to helping you connect with your spirit. Actually, I'm sure there aren't any "final" answers, because spiritual maturity is ever evolving. But I can assure you that nurturing your spirit is the most worthwhile step you can take toward achieving high performance health. Working on this step helps you work on the other nine steps to achieving high performance health. Connecting with your spirit will help you discover your purpose and direction. It may also enlighten your times of rest and provide a structure for establishing a third place. Certainly, connecting to your spirit is vital to discovering and living your spiritual age.

> I can assure you that nurturing your spirit is the most worthwhile step you can take toward achieving high performance health.

Connecting with your spirit is difficult and at times painful. But avoiding this process will prevent you from fully achieving high performance health.

TIPS:

- Recognize connecting with your spirit requires hard work and devote daily attention to it. Journaling can be a helpful practice.
- Record inspirational quotes in your daily tracker on your steps to achieving high performance health, and use this tracking process to nurture your spiritual health.
- Begin a regular course of reading that helps you explore connecting with your spirit. There are literally thousands of books available. Here are a few that have been meaningful to me:

  - Thomas Moore, *Care of the Soul*
  - M. Scott Peck, *The Road Less Traveled*
  - Kathleen Norris, *Dakota: A Spiritual Geography* and *Amazing Grace*
  - John Eldredge, *Wild at Heart: Discovering the Secret of a Man's Soul*
  - Henri Nouwen, *The Return of the Prodigal Son: A Story of Homecoming* and any other of his books
  - Anne Lamott, *Tender Mercies: Some Thoughts on Faith* and *Plan B: Further Thoughts on Faith*
  - Rick Warren, *The Purpose-Driven Life*

12 | A PERSONAL JOURNEY TO HIGH PERFORMANCE HEALTH

I shall be telling this with a sigh
Somewhere ages and ages hence:
Two roads diverged in a wood, and I—
I took the one less traveled by,
And that has made all the difference.

   —ROBERT FROST, "THE ROAD NOT TAKEN"

That feeling of safety you prize
Well, it comes at a hard hard price.

   —BRUCE SPRINGSTEEN, "HUMAN TOUCH"

As I began this book, I invited you to take my hands and join me on a journey. I close this book in much the same way, by sharing my own personal journey on the path toward high performance health.

Some years ago, I had the pleasure of meeting Nelson Mandela shortly after he was released from prison in South Africa. I was a young physician when he came to the United States after assuming the presidency of South

Africa. I must admit, I was still quite full of myself and proud of my accomplishments as a young physician. I was totally unprepared for what happened when I met Mr. Mandela. Here was a man who had spent more than twenty years of his life imprisoned in a small cell at Robin Island in South Africa, largely shut off from the outside world. But this terrible experience had not broken him. Instead, his spirit had grown deeper and stronger. He stood ramrod straight, despite his sixty-plus years, and emitted an aura of total awareness and total calm and total peace within himself. I was filled with awe and confusion. My pride in my accomplishments seemed empty. I wasn't ready in my own life to understand or in any way relate to the spiritual power this unique man possessed. But I was profoundly moved and humbled. Instinctively I knew my journey needed to continue, even if I didn't know just how.

My own journey toward spiritual health deepened with the birth of our first child. As a physician, I had the pleasure of delivering all of my children. (Actually, I did this in the company of an expert team of obstetricians. No cardiologist should be left alone to deliver babies, particularly his own!) When I first held Hart Elizabeth Rippe in my hands moments after her birth, and regarded her face, I knew for the first time that I had truly seen the face of God, that I could be forgiven, and that everything was going to be all right. Now, ten years and three daughters later, I consider myself the most blessed man alive. Not only have I fallen in love with a beautiful woman who helps me experience and fully appreciate the day-to-day blessings and joy of our life on this earth, but I continue to be touched, enlightened, and taught by four beautiful young daughters.

> Join me in making your life more than you ever thought possible.

I tell you this not because I believe I have a perfect life, but because I believe I have been given a chance to do more with my life than I ever dreamed possible. In the final analysis, that's what I am asking you to do in this book—to join me in making your life more than you ever thought possible.

Throughout this book, I have encouraged you to live fully and intentionally and keep track of your progress. So how am I doing on the path to high performance health? And how are you doing? Let me share with you a few thoughts.

I continue to work on discovering my life purpose and direction. I am very much at the beginning of this journey, but I have no doubt that the process is in full motion. I track it on a daily basis. I learned long ago that the discipline of writing down my thoughts and actions makes them much more coherent and overt. Making mind-body-spirit connections has not always been easy for me. As somebody who has always been physically active, I've found it easier to focus on my body than my mind, although I am much more diligent about the process than I have ever been before. I don't forget the inspiration of Nelson Mandela. How are you doing at tracking your goals and progress? At tapping the power of your mind-body-spirit connections?

What about the principles of active rest? I do take rest breaks throughout the day, although often they are designed to incorporate physical activity, since I find that active rest works best for me. I struggle with taking off one day a week and need to do better. Our vacations have turned into retreats from the world, whether they be active sporting vacations, such as skiing or wind surfing, or simply retreating to the country as a family to rediscover and reconnect with one another. Weekends are a more difficult challenge for me, since left to my own inclinations, I would work the whole time. Have you begun to make active rest a habit? To find what works for you?

I have established multiple third places. These have evolved from a health club to include the swimming pool and outdoor walking or jogging paths. But there is almost never a day when I do not visit a third place. It allows me my fifteen minutes of solitude, which I often incorporate into my thirty minutes of physical activity. It is not only a time when

I exercise my body but a time when I retreat from the world and experience the joy of true aloneness. What is your third place?

What about my spiritual and intellectual age? I am determined to continue to take on new intellectual endeavors, such as writing about subjects that challenge me. In fact, writing a book this personal would have been too daunting to try even five years ago. My children have been an enormous help and inspiration to me in pursuing a more youthful and more open spiritual age. In what ways are you nurturing your spiritual and intellectual life?

My eating habits are fairly good. It hasn't always been this way. Slowly, I have developed a nutritional pattern that closely mirrors what I have advised in step 8. I truly view the foods I choose and my eating patterns as critically important to fueling the level of performance that I desire and need in my life. I never miss breakfast. I typically consume a whole-grain cereal (oatmeal is my preference) along with a piece of fruit and an eight-ounce glass of orange

> I am convinced that the ten steps that I have described on the path toward high performance health are difficult but essential in getting the most out of life and fulfilling each of our destinies.

juice. I invariably have a cup of cappuccino (with low-fat milk, of course). Our family eats multiple servings of fish each week and consumes at least five servings of fruits and/or vegetables a day. We are not perfect, but we work very hard at our nutritional practices. Are you working on your nutritional practices?

My connection with others is a mixed bag. Stephanie and I have worked very hard on our connection to each other and our connection to our children. But this focus on our family has prevented us from giving time and attention to some of the friendships we value. My list of goals includes doing better in this area. How are you doing on your goals for connecting with others?

What about my connection to my spirit? It's a struggle. I have worked harder on this than any other aspect of my path toward high performance health. Looking inward and developing a trust in God have been both rewarding and challenging. I found Henri Nouwen's book *The Return of the Prodigal Son* particularly meaningful, as I also have struggled with the issues of being both a son and a father and developing the true belief that I am worthy of being found. What issues related to the care of your spirit and soul are you working on?

Why do I share these things about my journey and ask you about how you are progressing? Because I am convinced that the ten steps that I have described on the path toward high performance health are difficult but essential in getting the most out of life and fulfilling each of our destinies. I believe we learn from the experiences of others. I know I have learned from the experiences of many of my patients and hope that perhaps some of my own struggles in this area will prove helpful to you.

In the final analysis, I believe that moving along the path toward a new view of your health, as a high performance tool rather than the passive freedom from disease, boils down to the simple concept of learning to love yourself. One of my favorite poets, T. S. Eliot, describes this process more beautifully than I could ever hope to:

> Home is where one starts from. As we grow older
> The world becomes stranger, the pattern more complicated
> Of dead and living. Not the intense moment
> Isolated, with no before and after,
> But a lifetime burning in every moment
> And not the lifetime of one man only
> But of old stones that cannot be deciphered.
> There is a time for the evening under starlight,
> A time for the evening under lamplight
> (The evening with the photograph album).
> Love is most nearly itself

When here and now cease to matter.
Old men ought to be explorers
Here and there does not matter
We must be still and still moving
Into another intensity
For a further union, a deeper communion.
—T. S. Eliot, "East Coker," *The Four Quartets*[1]

In the end, each of us spends far too little time on this planet. It's up to us to make the most of that time to discover what Eliot describes as "a further union, a deeper communion." And the home where each of us starts is both physical and spiritual well-being and health. That is, in essence, what high performance health is all about—discovering that home and recognizing it for the first time.

I close with the words of my other favorite American poet, Robert Frost, from his famous poem "Stopping by Woods on a Snowy Evening."

The woods are lovely, dark, and deep,
But I have promises to keep,
And miles to go before I sleep,
And miles to go before I sleep.[2]

When I entered medicine twenty-five years ago, I made myself a promise to try to make the world healthier and a better place. I hope that I have made some contribution to this area and that this book represents a step along the way. The lives that we have been given are indeed "lovely, dark, and deep," and it's up to each of us to keep our promises before we sleep.

ABOUT THE AUTHOR

James M. Rippe, MD, is a graduate of Harvard College and Harvard Medical School with postgraduate training at Massachusetts General Hospital. He is the founder and director of the Rippe Lifestyle Institute, associate professor of medicine (Cardiology) at Tufts University School of Medicine, and professor of biomedical sciences at the University of Central Florida.

During the past twenty years, Dr. Rippe has established and run the largest research organization in the world, exploring how daily habits and actions impact short- and long-term health and quality of life. This organization, Rippe Lifestyle Institute, has published hundreds of studies that form the scientific basis for high performance health. Rippe Lifestyle Institute also conducts numerous studies every year on nutrition and healthy weight management.

Dr. Rippe is also the founder and director of the Rippe Health Assessment at Celebration Health, a series of comprehensive health evaluations for high performance individuals conducted at the state-of-the-art medical and fitness facility of Celebration Health in Orlando, Florida. Celebration Health is owned and operated by Florida Hospital, the largest hospital in America.

The author of thirty-six books, including fifteen health and fitness titles and twenty-one medical texts, Dr. Rippe wrote the best-selling book *The Rockport Walking Program* as well as three other walking books that won him the epithet "father of the modern American walking movement." Other books for general audiences include *The Exercise Exchange Program, Fit over Forty, Healthy Heart for Dummies, Heart Disease for Dummies, The Joint Health Prescription*, and *Weight Loss That Lasts*, written in collaboration with Weight Watchers International. His publishing has won him awards and numerous interviews on all broadcast network morning news programs, evening news, CNN, and top print media newspapers and magazines.

Dr. Rippe edits the major intensive-care textbook in the United States, *Irwin and Rippe's Intensive Care Medicine*, which is used in virtually every intensive care unit in the United States. He also edits *Lifestyle Medicine*, the only comprehensive textbook and academic journal on lifestyle medicine, as well as *The American Journal of Lifestyle Medicine*, the only academic peer-reviewed journal in this area. Dr. Rippe also serves as a leader of a variety of associations and boards and has received numerous awards.

A lifelong and avid athlete, Dr. Rippe is regarded as one of the leading authorities on preventive cardiology, health, fitness, and healthy weight loss in the United States. He lives outside of Boston with his wife, television news anchor Stephanie Hart, and their four children.

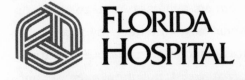

FLORIDA HOSPITAL

AMERICA'S TRUSTED LEADER FOR HEALTH AND HEALING

For nearly one hundred years the mission of Florida Hospital has been to help our patients, guests and friends achieve whole-person health and healing. With seven hospital campuses and sixteen walk-in medical centers, Florida Hospital cares for over one million patients every year.

Over a decade ago Florida Hospital began working with the Disney Corporation to create a groundbreaking facility that would showcase the model of healthcare for the twenty-first century and stay on the cutting edge of medical technology as it develops. Working with a team of medical experts, industry leaders, and healthcare futurists, we designed and built a whole-person health hospital named Celebration Health located in Disney's town of Celebration, Florida. Since opening its doors in 1997, Celebration Health has been awarded the *Premier Patient Services Innovator Award* as "The Model for Healthcare Delivery in the 21st Century."

When Dr. Lydia Parmele, the first female physician in the state of Florida, and her medical team opened our first healthcare facility in 1908, their goal was to create a healing environment where they not only treated illness, but also provided the support and education necessary to help patients achieve whole-person health mentally, physically, spiritually, emotionally, and socially.

215

The lifestyle advocated by our founders remains central to all we do at Florida Hospital. We teach patients how to reduce the risk of disease through healthy lifestyle choices, encouraging the use of natural remedies such as fresh air, sunshine, water, rest, nutrition, exercise, outlook, faith, and interpersonal relationships.

Today, Florida Hospital:

- Ranks number one in the nation for inpatient admissions by the American Hospital Association.
- Is the largest provider of Medicare services in the country.
- Ranks number one in the nation for number of heart procedures performed each year. MSNBC named Florida Hospital "America's Heart Hospital".
- Operates many nationally recognized centers of excellence including Cardiology, Cancer, Orthopedics, Neurology & Neurosurgery, Digestive Disorders and Minimally Invasive Surgery.
- Is one of the "Top 10 Best Places in the Country to have a Baby" according to *Fit Pregnancy* magazine.

For more information about Florida Hospital and our other whole-person health products, including books, music, videos, conferences, seminars, and other resources, please contact us at:

Florida Hospital Publishing
683 Winyah Drive, Orlando, FL 32803
Phone: 407-303-7711   Fax: 407-303-1818
Email: healthproducts@flhosp.org
www.FloridaHospital.com   www.CreationHealth.com

APPENDIX

In addition to the resources in this appendix, check our website, www.highperformancehealth.net, for many more.

HIGH PERFORMANCE HEALTH WALKING PROGRAM

The High Performance Health Walking Program's easy-to-use calendar takes you from sedentary to physically fit in 20 weeks. If you are already somewhat active, you can start at your level. You can also adapt the program to other physical activities: I give you tips below the calendar.

EQUIPMENT NEEDED: Walking shoes. Comfortable, weather-appropriate clothing. Stick-to-it promise to yourself.

HOW TO USE THE CALENDAR

    1. *Start slow.* If you have not been following a formal program of activity, I recommend that you start with week 1. If you are already walking regularly, pick the week level that matches your current activity and try it. You can move forward or back as needed.

    2. *Intensity.* The first column lists the intensity level for each week's walk. "Light" indicates a walking pace that is faster than a stroll, but does not "push" you; this pace is probably close to your normal,

everyday pace. "Moderate" intensity is a notch or two above "light"; your breathing and perception of exertion are increased, but you should be able to talk normally. "Brisk" is a notch or two above "moderate"; your breathing rate and perception of exertion are elevated but you should not be breathless.

3. *Warm up and cool down.* Always begin your walk (or activity session) by warming up and end it by cooling down. To warm up simply walk at a "light" pace for 3-4 minutes and cool down the same way.

HIGH PERFORMANCE HEALTH WALKING PROGRAM

Week	Intensity	Mon.	Tues.	Wed.	Thurs.	Fri.	Sat.	Sun.
1	light	10 min		10 min		10 min		
2	light-mod	10 min		10 min		10 min		
3	light-mod	12 min		12 min		12 min	(10 min)*	
4	moderate	12 min		12 min		12 min	(12 min)	
5	moderate	15 min		12 min		15 min	(12 min)	
6	moderate	15 min		15 min		15 min		(15 min)
7	mod-brisk	15 min		15 min	(12 min)	15 min		
8	mod-brisk	15 min		15min		15 min	15 min	
9	mod-brisk	18 min		18 min		18 min		15 min
10	brisk	15 min		18 min		18 min	15 min	
11	brisk	18 min		18 min		18 min		18 min
12	brisk	20 min		18 min		20 min		18 min
13	brisk	20 min		20 min	(15 min)	20 min		20 min
14	brisk	20 min		22 min		20 min	22 min	
15	brisk	22 min		22 min	(20 min)	22 min		22min
16	brisk	25 min		22 min		25 min	(20 min)	22 min
17	brisk	25 min		25 min	20 min	25 min		25 min
18	brisk	25 min		27 min		25 min		27 min
19	brisk	27 min	(25 min)	30 min		27 min		30 min
20	brisk	30 min		30 min	30 min	30 min		30 min

* All sessions in parentheses ( ) are optional.

You may vary days of the week for walk sessions; simply maintain the pattern of the calendar. To increase sessions duration beyond 30 minutes, continue gradually increasing minutes.

USING THE HIGH PERFORMANCE HEALTH WALKING PROGRAM FOR OTHER ACTIVITIES. For variety you may choose to alternate other activities such as cycling or swimming with walking. Or perhaps you prefer an alternate primary activity. Here are tips for adapting the calendar.

Cycling (stationary indoor)—use the same duration for sessions, gradually increase the resistance setting to simulate moderate to brisk pace.

Cycling (outdoor)—cycling on level terrain, increase times by five minutes

—cycling on hilly terrain, decrease times by five minutes or take 1 minute breaks within the session as needed

Swimming—use the same duration, but to begin do not try to swim 10 minutes continuously. Swim 5 minutes, rest 1, swim five. Increase the duration of your continuous swim gradually. Repeat a week's pattern as necessary. Recommended stroke for fitness swimming: freestyle. You may also vary strokes.

Treadmills—Treadmills vary widely in the features they offer. Use the times of the training calendar, gradually increase either the speed or incline each week to maintain the level of intensity indicated.

Elliptical trainers—Elliptical trainers vary widely in the features they offer. Use the times of the training calendar, gradually increase either resistance or incline each week to maintain the level of intensity indicated.

Rowing & ski machines—Decrease the time by five minutes per session or take rest breaks as with swimming. Repeat each week's level twice.

Jogging—Jogging is a high impact activity that can stress your joints. Use properly fitted running shoes. Do not begin jogging until you can briskly walk 30 minutes on 4 or 5 days a week. Begin jogging gradually. I recommend beginning by jogging for 1 minute (or 100 hundred steps), then walking 2 minutes (200 steps). Gradually add time or steps to the jogging component. Continue to take walking breaks as needed. Do not run through pain.

What about stretching and weight training activities? Building flexibility and strength can be very important to building high performance health. I provide short stretching and strength training routines on our website: www.highperformancehealth.net.

OUTLINE FOR YOUR MEDICAL HISTORY

Before a first visit to a new physician or specialist, it's helpful to gather the following information in an accessible form.

1. If you are seeing a specialist, what is the name and address of your primary physician.
2. Do you have your health insurance information?
3. What is purpose for the visit? Describe your concern or condition.
4. What health conditions or medical problems do you currently have? Are you under the care of a physician or taking medication for these.
5. What health conditions or medical problems have you had in the past?
6. What medications do you currently take?
   Prescription?
   Over-the-counter?
   Nutritional supplements?
7. Have you ever been hospitalized? For what illness or problem? When?
8. Have you ever had surgery? For what condition? When?
9. Do you have allergies to any foods or medicines? Environmental conditions?

10. Describe your physical activity program or estimate your level of physical activity.

11. What is your family medical history? Did your mother or father have any chronic conditions such as heart disease or high blood pressure? Cancer? Any other members of your immediate

If you are being referred to a specialist, ask the referring physician if there are any records or test results that you should take to the specialist.

RECOMMENDED RESOURCES

In addition to the following online resources, see our website: www.highperformancehealth.net, for additional recommendations of useful resources on the Web and in print.

GOVERNMENT GENERAL HEALTH AND MEDICAL INFORMATION

http://medlineplus.gov (National Library of Medicine)
http://health.nih.gov (National Institutes of Health)
www.healthfinder.gov (National Health Information Service)
www.cdc.gov (Centers for Disease Control and Prevention)
www.fitness.gov (President's Council on Physical Fitness and Sports)
www.MyPyramid.gov (Dietary Guidelines for Americans 2005)
www.nutrition.gov (U.S. Department of Agriculture)

HEATH-CARE ASSOCIATIONS OR AGENCIES

http://familydoctor.org (American Academy of Family Physicians)
www.ama-assn.org (American Medical Association)
www.americanheart.org (American Heart Association)
www.lungusa.org (American Lung Association)
www.cancer.org (American Cancer Society)
www.eatright.org (American Dietetic Association)

www.arthritisfoundation.org (Arthritis Foundation)

www.getactiveamerica.com (International Health, Racquet, and Sportsclub Association)

COMMERCIAL SITES

www.webmd.com

www.mayoclinic.com

www.floridahospital.com

www.rippehealth.com

www.getbpdown.com

www.drugs.com

www.supplementwatch.com

www.weightwatchers.com

NOTES

CHAPTER 1

1. "Prevalence Statistics Related to Overweight and Obesity" from Weight Control Information Network of NIDDK of National Institutes of Health. http://win.niddk.nih.gov/statistics/index.htm#preval.

2. "Adult Cigarette Smoking in the United States: Current Estimates Fact Sheet," November 2006. CDC, National Center for Chronic Disease Prevention and Health Promotion, Tobacco Information and Prevention Source. http://www.cdc.gov/tobacco/factsheets/ AdultCigaretteSmoking_FactSheet.htm

3. "Physical Activity and Fitness" from Healthy People 2010. http://www.healthypeople.gov/Document/HTML/Volume2/ 22Physical.htm#_Toc490380795. "For individuals who do not engage in any physical activity during their leisure time, taking the first step toward developing a pattern of regular physical activity is important. Unfortunately, few individuals engage in regular physical activity despite its documented benefits. Only about 23 percent of adults in the United States report regular, vigorous physical activity that involves large muscle groups in dynamic movement for 20 minutes or longer 3 or more days per week. Only 15 percent of adults report physical activity for 5 or more days per week for 30 minutes or longer, and another 40 percent do not participate in any regular physical activity."

4. Data from Behavioral Risk Factor Surveillance System (CDC) summarized on www.5aday.org.

5. Meir J. Stampfer, FB Hu, J.E .Manson, E.B. Rimm, and W.C. Willett, "Primary Prevention of Coronary Heart Disease in Women Through

Diet and Lifestyle," *New England Journal of Medicine* 343(1), (6 July 2000):16–22.

6. Ibid.

CHAPTER 2

Epigraph   "Hymn of Promise" by Natalie Sleeth © 1986 Hope Publishing Company. Carol Stream, IL 60188. All rights reserved. Used by permission.

1. Excerpt from "Little Gidding" in *Four Quartets*, copyright 1942 by T.S. Eliot and renewed by Esme Valerie Eliot, reprinted by permission of Harcourt, Inc.

2. "Hymn of Promise" by Natalie Sleeth. Used by permission.

CHAPTER 3

1. R.R. Pate, M. Pratt, S.N. Blair, W.L Haskell, C.A. Macera, C. Bouchard, et al. "Physical Activity and Public Health: A Recommendation From the Centers for Disease Control and Prevention and the American College of Sports Medicine," *Journal of the American Medical Association* 273 (1995):402–407.

2. U.S. Department of Health and Human Services, *Physical Activity and Health: A Report of the Surgeon General.* Atlanta, GA: U.S. Department of Health and Human Services, Centers for Disease Control and Prevention, National Center for Chronic Disease Prevention and Health Promotion, 1996.

3. Paul Taylor, Cary Funk, and Peyton Craighill, "Americans See Weight Problems Everywhere But in the Mirror," *Peyton Research Center, A Social Trends Report,* 11 April 2006. http://pewresearch.org/assets/social/pdf/Obesity.pdf.

4. R. R. Pate, et al.

5. "Prevalence Statistics Related to Overweight and Obesity" from Weight Control Information Network of NIDDK of National Institutes of Health. http://win.niddk.nih.gov/statistics/index.htm#preval.

6. James M. Rippe, M.D. and Weight Watchers. *Weight Loss That Lasts: Break Through the 10 Big Diet Myths.* New Jersey: John Wiley & Sons, Inc, 2005.

7. H.R. Wyatt, G.K. Grunwald, C.L. Mosca, M.L. Klem, R.R. Wing, and J.O. Hill. "Long-term weight loss and breakfast in subjects in the

National Weight Control Registry", *Obesity Research* 10(2), (February 2002): 78–82.

8. The Surgeon General's Report on Nutrition and Health, 1988. www.surgeongeneral.gov/library/reports.htm. Latest data can be found on www.cdc.gov/nchs/fastats/lcod.htm.

9. U.S. Department of Health and Human Services, U.S. Department of Agriculture Dietary Guidelines for Americans 2005. 6th edition. Washington, D.C.: U.S. Government Printing Office, January 2005. www.healthierus.gov/guidelines.

10. "Health habits of U.S. adults, 1985: the "Alameda 7" revisited." *Public Health Reports* 1986 Nov–Dec;101 (6):571–80.

11. Robert Frost, "The Road Not Taken" found in *The Poetry of Robert Frost* (New York: Holt, 1969).

CHAPTER 4

1. R.B. Case, A.J. Moss, N. Case, M. McDermott, and S. Eberly, "Living Alone After Myocardial Infarction," *JAMA* 267, (1992): 515–519.

2. For more information see www.cdc.gov/HealthyYouth/ physicalactivity/promoting_health/.

3. John Eldredge, *Wild at Heart: Discovering the Secret of a Man's Soul* (Nashville: Thomas Nelson, 2006).

4. Henri Nouwen, *The Return of the Prodigal Son* (New York: Image, a division of Doubleday, 1994).

5. Ellen J. Langer, *Mindfulness* (New York: Addison Wesley, 1990).

6. For more information see Stanford Heart Disease Prevention Program at http://prevention.stanford.edu/default.asp.

CHAPTER 5

1. Jack Nicklaus and Ken Bowden, *Golf My Way* (New York: Simon & Schuster, 1998).

2. Monica Reed and Donna K. Wallace, *The Creation Health Breakthrough: 8 Essentials to Revolutionize Your Health Physically, Mentally and Spiritually* (New York: Hatchette, 2007).

3. Richard Leider and David Shapiro, *Repacking Your Bags* (San Francisco: Berrett-Koehler, 2002).

4. James Montgomery, "Prayer is the Soul's Sincere Desire," © 1818.

5. T.L. Saudia, M.R. Kinney, K.C. Brown, and L. Young-Ward, "Health

Locus of Control and Helpfulness of Prayer," *Heart Lung* 20(1),
(January 1991):60–5. www.ncbi.nlm.nih.gov/entrez/
query.fcgi?db=pubmed&cmd=Retrieve&dopt=AbstractPlus&list_uids=
1988394&query_hl=72&itool=pubmed_docsum.

6. Ken Pelletier, MD., *Mind As Healer, Mind As Slayer: A Holistic Approach to Preventing Stress Disorders* (New York: Peter Smith Publisher, 1984).

CHAPTER 6

Epigraph John Berryman, *The Dream Songs.* (New York: Farrar, Straus and Giroux, 1982).

1. S. Das and J.H. O'Keefe. "Behavioral Cardiology: Recognizing and Addressing the Profound Impact of Psychosocial Stress on Cardiovascular Health," *Current Atherosclerosis Reports* 8(2), (March 2006): 111–8.

2. For an excellent discussion of the relevant research, see Dr. Redford and Dr. Virginia Williams' book, *Anger Kills* (New York: Harper, 1998).

3. David Spiegel, JR Bloom, HC Kraemer, and E. Gottheil, "Effect of Psychosocial Treatment on Survival of Patients with Metastatic Breast Cancer," *Lancet* 2(8668), (14 October 1989): 888–91.

4. American Psychological Association APA Help Center "How Does Stress Affect Us?" www.apahelpcenter.org/articles/article.php?id=11.

5. Jon Kabat-Zinn , *Wherever You Go, There You Are: Mindfulness Meditation in Everyday Life* (New York: Hyperion, 2005). *Full Catastrophe Living: Using the Wisdom of Your Body and Mind to Face Stress, Pain, and Illness* (New York: Delta, 1990).

6. Williams, *Anger Kills.*

7. Ibid.

8. "Human Touch" by Bruce Springsteen. Copyright © 1992 Bruce Springsteen (ASCAP). Reprinted by permission. International copyright secured. All rights reserved.

9. Rad Smith, *Distant Early Warning* (Dorset, VT: Tupelo Press, 2005).

10. Redford B. Williams, J.C. Barefoot, R.M. Califf, T.L. Haney, W.B. Saunders, D.B. Pryor, M.A. Hlatky, I.C. Siegler, and D.B. Mark, "Prognostic Importance of Social and Economic Resources Among Medically Treated Patients with Angiographically Documented Coronary Artery Disease," *JAMA.* (22–29 January 1992), 267(4):520–4.

11. Thomas Moore, *Care of the Soul* (New York: Harper, 1994).
12. Martin Luther King Jr., Speech in Detroit, June 23, 1963.
13. Henri Nouwen, *The Return of the Prodigal Son* (New York: Continuum International Publishing Group, 1996).
14. Excerpt from "Little Gidding" in *Four Quartets*, copyright 1942 by T.S. Eliot and renewed by Esme Valerie Eliot, reprinted by permission of Harcourt, Inc.
15. Pirkko L.Graves, et al., "Psychological Predictors of Mortality: Evidence from a 41–Year Prospective Study," March 1991. www.jhu.edu/~jhumag/0601web/study.html.
16. L.G. Russek and G.E.Schwartz, "Perceptions of Parental Caring Predict Health Status in Midlife: A 35-year follow-up of the Harvard Mastery of Stress Study," *Psychosomatic Medicine*, 59(2), (March/April 1997):144–9.

CHAPTER 7

1. Jared Sandberg, "Why Multitasking Doesn't Work," *Wall Street Journal.* (September 13, 2006). Found on http://www.careerjournal.com/columnists/cubicleculture/20060913-cubicle.html.
2. "Insomnia: Assessment and Management in Primary Care National Center on Sleep Disorders Research" found on http://www.nhlbi.nih.gov/about/ncsdr/index.htm.
3. Daniel W. Nixon, MD., *The Cancer Recovery Eating Plan: The Right Foods to Help Fuel Your Recovery* (New York: Three Rivers Press, a division of Random House, 1996).
4. Bernie Siegel, MD. *Love, Medicine and Miracles: Lessons Learned about Self-Healing from a Surgeon's Experience with Exceptional Patients* (New York: Harper, 1990). Bernie Siegel, MD *Peace, Love and Healing: Bodymind Communication & the Path to Self-Healing: An Exploration* (New York: Harper, 1990).
5. "Obesity: A Global Epidemic" found on http://www.obesity.org/subs/fastfacts/obesity_global_epidemic.shtml.
6. James M. Rippe, MD and Weight Watchers, *Weight Watchers Weight Loss That Lasts: Break Through the 10 Big Diet Myths* (Hoboken, NJ: Wiley Press, 2005).
7. Salyn Boles, "1 Out of 3 Adults Has High Blood Pressure," August 23, 2004 found on http://www.webmd.com/content/article/93/102119.htm.

8. James M. Rippe, MD, *The Joint Health Prescription* (Darby, PA: Diane Publishing, 2004).
9. "What Problems Are Caused by Smoking?" found on http://www.answers.com/topic/smoking.
10. John W. Farquhar and Gene A. Spiller, *The Last Puff: Ex-Smokers Share the Secrets of Their Success* (New York: W. W. Norton & Company, 1991).

CHAPTER 8

1. For more information visit the American Cancer Society at www.cancer.org.
2. Eugenia E. Calle, Ph.D., Carmen Rodriguez, M.D., M.P.H., Kimberly Walker-Thurmond, B.A., and Michael J. Thun, M.D, "Overweight, Obesity, and Mortality from Cancer in a Prospectively Studied Cohort of U.S. Adults," *JAMA* 348:1625–1638 (24 April 2006):17.
3. James O. Prochaska, John Norcross, and Carlo DiClemente, *Changing for Good* (New York: William Morrow, 1994). Reprinted by permission of HarperCollins Publishers.

CHAPTER 9

Epigraph   Marion Wright Edelman, *The Measure of Our Success* (New York: Harper, 1993).
1. Dr. Jim Loeher and Tony Schwartz, *The Power of Full Engagement: Managing Energy, Not Time, Is the Key to High Performance and Personal Renewal* (New York: Free Press, a division of Simon and Schuster, 2003).
2. Max Depree, *Leadership Is an Art* (New York: Currency Books, a division of Doubleday, 2004).
3. Carl R. Rogers, *On Becoming a Person* (London: Constable and Co, 1990).

CHAPTER 10

Epigraph   Viktor E. Frankl, *Man's Search for Meaning*. Copyright © 1959, 1962, 1984, 1992 by Viktor E. Frankl. Reprinted by permission of Beacon Press, Boston.
1. Timothy Egan, "The Rise of Shrinking-Vacation Syndrome," *The New York Times*, 20 August 2006. http://travel2.nytimes.com/2006/08/20/us/20vacation.html?pagewanted=print.

2. Frankl, *Man's Search for Meaning.*

3. Henri Nouwen, *The Return of the Prodigal Son* (New York: Image, a division of Doubleday, 1994).

4. Thomas Moore, *The Care of the Soul* (New York: Harper, 1994).

5. Marilynne Robinson, *Gilead* (New York: Farrar, Straus, and Giroux, 2006).

CHAPTER 11

1. Dorothy and Jerome Singer, *The House of Make Believe: Children's Play and the Developing Imagination* (Cambridge, MA: Harvard University Press, 1992).

2. Jane Brody, "Take Care of the Body, It's the Temple of the Mind" accessed on http://www.research.cornell.edu/VPR/CWC171-03/pdfs/commentary.pdf.

CHAPTER 12

Epigraph   Robert Frost, "The Road Not Taken" found in *The Poetry of Robert Frost* (New York: Holt, 1969).

1. Excerpt from "East Coker" in *Four Quartets*, copyright 1942 by T.S. Eliot and renewed by Esme Valerie Eliot, reprinted by permission of Harcourt, Inc.

2. Frost, *The Poetry of Robert Frost.*

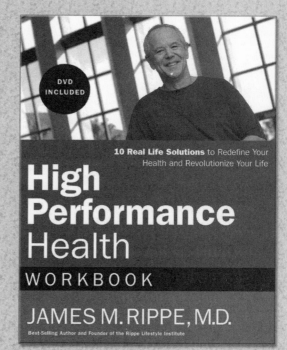
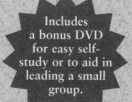
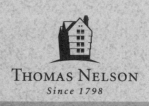